Comments on **Stroke – the 'at your fingertips' guide**
from readers

'If you buy only one book about stroke, it should be *Stroke: the 'at your fingertips' guide*. It is an excellent information resource, easily accessible and written by experts. Whether you are a stroke survivor, friend or family member, a carer, or a health professional working in the stroke field, you'll find useful information in this book.'

Jon Barrick BSc MCIH MBA FCMI
Chief Executive, The Stroke Association

'It is an excellent and long overdue book, which will be of interest not only to stroke survivors and their carers but also to health-care professionals of all disciplines. It is not too technical and explains things simply without being patronising.'

Donal O'Kelly,
Former Director, Different Strokes

'It's a good read, covering all of the usual questions people ask. Congratulations to the authors.'

Eoin M Redahan,
Former Director of Public Relations,
The Stroke Association

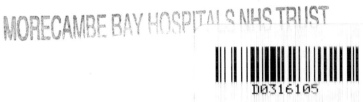

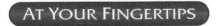

STROKE

THE COMPREHENSIVE AND MEDICALLY ACCURATE MANUAL ABOUT STROKE AND HOW TO DEAL WITH IT

Anthony Rudd MA MB BChir FRCP (London)
Consultant Stroke Physician, Guy's and St Thomas' Hospital, London
Programme Director (Stroke), Clinical Effectiveness
and Evaluation Unit, Royal College of Physicians, London
President, British Association of Stroke Physicians

Penny Irwin RGN MSc
Clinical Effectiveness Facilitator, Clinical Effectiveness Unit,
Royal College of Physicians, London

Bridget Penhale CQSW
Senior Lecturer in Gerontology, University of Sheffield

CLASS PUBLISHING • LONDON

Text © Dr Anthony Rudd, Penny Irwin and Bridget Penhale 2000, 2005
Typography © Class Publishing (London) Ltd 2000, 2005

Printing history
First published 2000
Second edition 2005
Reprinted 2006

616.81
RUD

The authors and publisher welcome feedback from the users of this book.
Please contact the publishers.

Class Publishing (London) Ltd
Barb House, Barb Mews, London W6 7PA
Telephone: 020 7371 2119
Fax: 020 7371 2878 [International +4420]
Email: post@class.co.uk

The information presented in this book is accurate and current to the best of
the authors' knowledge. The authors and publisher, however, make no
guarantee as to, and assume no responsibility for, the correctness, sufficiency
or completeness of such information or recommendation. The reader is
advised to consult a doctor regarding all aspects of individual health care.

A CIP catalogue record for this book is available from the British Library.

ISBN 1 85959 113 2

10 9 8 7 6 5 4 3 2

Edited by Gillian Clarke
Indexed by Val Elliston
Cartoons by Jane Taylor
Typeset by Martin Bristow
Printed and bound in Finland by WS Bookwell, Juva

Contents

Acknowledgements   ix

Introduction   1

CHAPTER 1 **What is a stroke?**   3
What happens with a stroke?   6
Getting better   13
Not getting better?   19

CHAPTER 2 **The first few days**   23
Investigations   24
Treatment   29
Rehabilitation issues   38

CHAPTER 3 **Getting moving again**   51
Physiotherapy   52
Muscle stiffness or weakness   57
Aids and equipment   61
Wheelchairs   64
Complementary therapies   67

CHAPTER 4 **Swallowing and nutrition**   68
Swallowing   69
Nutrition and diet   75

CHAPTER 5 *Speech and language*   86
Problems understanding and speaking   87
Other problems   88
Speech and language therapy   92

CHAPTER 6 *Personal care*   96
Incontinence   97
Constipation   103
Skin care   104

CHAPTER 7 *Memory, mood and sleep*   108
Memory   109
Mood   112
Sleep   118

CHAPTER 8 *Pain and sensation*   122
Pain   123
Sensation   129

CHAPTER 9 *The senses*   132
Vision   133
Taste and smell   136
Hearing and balance   136

CHAPTER 10 *Living with disability*   138
Occupational therapy   140
Aids and equipment at home   142
Emotional factors   144

CHAPTER 11 *Why have I had a stroke and what can
          I do to prevent another one?*   146
Risk factors for stroke   147
Drugs to prevent stroke   164

Surgery to prevent stroke 172
Developing new symptoms 174

CHAPTER 12 *Discharge from hospital* 177
Managing at home 178
Moving in with the family 184
Moving into sheltered housing 186
Moving into a care home 187
Miscellaneous 193

CHAPTER 13 *Relationships* 195
Sexual matters 196
Family planning 201
Help for family carers 202
When a partner is in a care home 208

CHAPTER 14 *Leisure, work and money* 211
Leisure 212
Work 215
Money 217

CHAPTER 15 *Research and future developments* 221
Research projects 222
The future 223

GLOSSARY 227

APPENDIX 1 Useful addresses 233

APPENDIX 2 Useful publications 247

INDEX 249

Acknowledgements

We are grateful to all the people who have helped in the production of this book, and in particular we thank the following for their contributions and support:

> Jon Barrick and The Stroke Association
> Christina Meacham and Different Strokes
> Juliet MacKellaig and Lorna McTernan of Chest, Heart &
>   Stroke Scotland
> Lucy Matsas
> Ken and Helen Cutting
> Suzanne Marsello
> Johnathan Potter
> Ian Starke

And, of course, the people who provided us with the questions that form the basis of this book.

Any errors are our own.

MORECAMBE BAY HOSPITALS NHS TRUST

Introduction

If you have recently had a stroke, you will be one of about 130,000 people in the UK this year to have suffered a similar fate. That is a stroke happening to someone new every five minutes. At any one time in an average district general hospital there will be between 20 and 30 people occupying beds as a result of stroke. It is the fourth commonest cause of death and the most frequent cause of disability in adults. At any one time there are 350,000 people living with the long-term disability that sometimes results from stroke. It affects people of all ages, including children, although half of all cases occur in those over 75 years of age.

The life of every person who has a stroke will change, even if they make a full recovery. The effects of stroke are not limited to that individual: family, friends and carers will also be affected. Society as a whole suffers. Every year around 25,000 people of working age have a stroke. The NHS spends 4% of its budget providing care for people with stroke, and a considerable proportion of spending by social services goes to providing continuing support for people at home and in residential care.

Yet, despite the importance of the condition to individuals and society, only recently has much attention been paid to it by research scientists, the medical profession or the politicians. It still receives only a tiny proportion of funding compared with the money spent on cancer research and it is only now that a speciality of 'stroke medicine' is being developed. A recent audit has shown that many areas of the UK do not offer the sort of care that people with stroke deserve. So, if you (or a relative) have had a stroke, it is vital that you know as much about the illness as possible. You should know what has happened to you and what treatment you have a right to expect to receive. Services are slowly improving, but they will improve much more quickly if you demand your rights.

In this book we answer, as frankly as we can, many of the questions that we have been asked by people over the years. In some instances the honest answer is 'we don't know'. Foremost among these difficult questions is 'how much recovery will I make and how long will it take?' Hopefully, in a few years' time there will be fewer occasions when the answer is a shrug of the shoulders. One of the key messages we hope to put across is not to be shy about approaching the doctors, nurses, therapists and social workers involved in your care. They are there to provide you with a service, and should be happy to sit down with you and explain what is happening. The information provided by The Stroke Association (in England and Wales), Chest, Heart & Stroke Scotland, Northern Ireland Chest, Heart & Stroke Association and Different Strokes will also be useful.

We have tried to avoid using medical jargon but it is inevitable that some terms must be mentioned. In such instances they are explained briefly at their first mention but they are also listed in a Glossary at the back of the book in case you want to refresh your memory about what they mean.

What is a stroke?

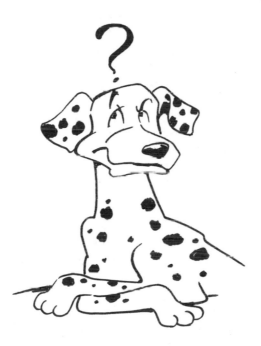

The brain is split into two halves, the left and the right *hemi-spheres*. At the base of the brain is the *cerebellum* and leading from the brain down into the spinal cord is the *brainstem*. All the information that is detected by the nerve endings in the body is passed up the spinal cord and brainstem to one of the cerebral hemispheres. There the brain decides what it needs to do and sends the relevant instructions back down the same route to activate the muscles. For example, if you touch something very hot, your brain receives the message and tells your hand to move away. Figure 1 is a simplified diagram of the main parts of the brain.

The left hemisphere largely controls the right-hand side of the body, and the right hemisphere the left side. The brain has specific parts devoted to specific functions (see Figure 2). For example, the language areas are usually in the left-hand side of the brain, except in a small proportion of left-handed people in whom the language area is on the right. The areas processing information about vision are at the back of the brain. Control of muscle and sensory function is situated near the front of the brain in the *frontal* and *parietal lobes*, and co-ordination is controlled by the cerebellum.

The blood to the brain travels from the heart through the aorta (the main artery from the heart) and then into one of four arteries

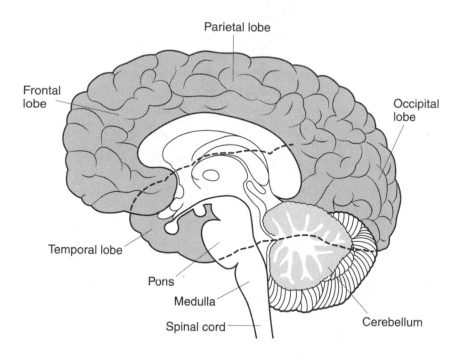

Figure 1 The main parts of the brain (viewed from the side)

that lead to the brain. At the front are the two carotid arteries that you can feel pulsating in your neck, either side of the windpipe, and at the back, running alongside the vertebral column (the spine), are the two vertebral arteries. Once the four arteries have entered the skull, they are linked together in the *circle of Willis*

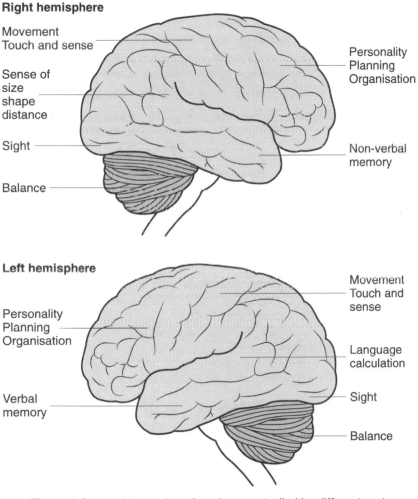

Figure 2 Some of the various functions controlled by different parts of the brain

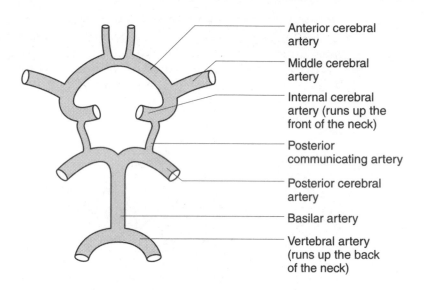

Anterior cerebral artery

Middle cerebral artery

Internal cerebral artery (runs up the front of the neck)

Posterior communicating artery

Posterior cerebral artery

Basilar artery

Vertebral artery (runs up the back of the neck)

Figure 3 The blood supply to the brain, including the 'circle of Willis'

(see Figure 3). This is a very important anatomical feature, because, if one artery is blocked, sometimes there is enough blood provided from the other arteries joining the circle to prevent major damage being done. Leading off the circle of Willis are the six major cerebral arteries – anterior, middle and posterior (one of each on either side), supplying respectively the front, middle and back parts of the brain (see Figure 4). Any of these can be blocked, causing a stroke, but the commonest to be affected is the middle cerebral artery.

What happens with a stroke?

What actually is a stroke?

A stroke is what happens when the brain is damaged as the result of a problem with its blood supply. Each part of the brain is responsible for a particular function, so the symptoms that result

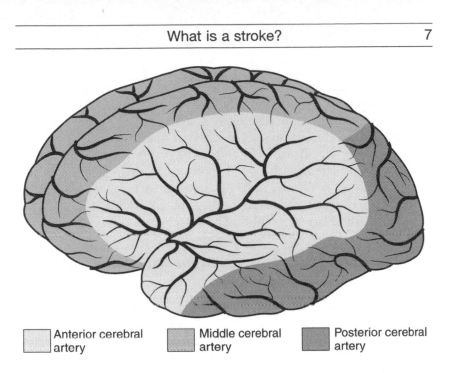

Anterior cerebral
artery

Middle cerebral
artery

Posterior cerebral
artery

Figure 4 The areas of the brain supplied by the cerebral arteries

will depend on which part of the brain is deprived of its blood supply.

By noting down exactly what the problems are and examining you, it is usually possible for the doctor to be reasonably accurate in identifying where the stroke is. Strokes can be large or small, depending on which artery and which part of it has been affected. The damage can occur in two major ways. The commonest, occurring in about 80% of cases, is where one of the arteries becomes blocked with a blood clot. This can be due to 'furring up' of the artery with cholesterol, which results in the lining of the artery becoming rough and allowing blood cells and *platelets* to stick to it. (Platelets are the fragments in the blood that stick together when necessary to form a blood clot.) Alternatively, a clot can be formed further downstream, then becoming dislodged and travelling up the artery until it reaches a point where the clot is bigger than the artery, where it becomes stuck. These clots can come from the heart or the aorta (the main artery from the heart) or from the carotid or vertebral arteries. The blockage causes the part of the brain supplied by that artery to be deprived of oxygen and nourishment, resulting in damage to the nerve cells.

The remaining 20% of strokes are due to haemorrhage (bleeding) into the brain – *intracerebral haemorrhage* – or onto the surface of the brain – *subarachnoid haemorrhage*. Intracerebral haemorrhage can occur from any of the arteries in the brain, but most commonly affects small arteries deep inside the brain. A haemorrhage causes damage as a result of the escaped blood squashing the surrounding brain tissue.

My brother, who had a stroke a while back, reckons that I have had a TIA. What is that?

'TIA' is the abbreviation for 'transient ischaemic attack' – which can be very frightening. It is exactly the same as a stroke except that, if you have a TIA, you will recover completely from it within 24 hours. As with a stroke, it can cause many different symptoms, depending on which part of the brain is affected. One special type of TIA is called *amaurosis fugax*. This is where the artery to the eye becomes temporarily blocked, resulting in loss of vision. People who have had such an attack often describe the sensation as being like a curtain coming down in front of the eye.

TIAs should be treated seriously, and you should see your doctor as soon as possible. He or she will probably start you on aspirin immediately and should refer you on to a specialist for some further tests. You should regard a TIA as a warning sign that all is not right with the blood supply to your brain. If the appropriate treatment is given, you might never have another one, but if it is ignored you are at a greater risk of having a full-blown stroke. It is important to act quickly when you have symptoms that might be due to a TIA. The greatest risk of going on to develop a stroke is within the first few weeks. It is therefore important that you are referred to a specialist, seen and investigated as soon as possible.

The latest National Guidelines for stroke recommend that someone with a TIA is seen by a specialist, investigated and receives appropriate treatment within seven days of the symptoms. Unfortunately, in many parts of the world that will be regarded as unachievable. Nevertheless, it has been achieved for people with chest pain that might progress to a heart attack, so why should TIA and stroke be treated differently?

What is a mini-stroke?

'Mini-stroke' is the term that is sometimes given to a mild stroke that recovers very quickly, although not as quickly as a TIA. The advice given for TIA in the answer above is equally true for mini-strokes. Seek medical attention as quickly as possible.

My doctor has told me that I have had a haemorrhage in the brain. What does this mean?

About one in five of all strokes that happen in the UK is due to cerebral haemorrhage. When a hole forms in the wall of an artery in the brain, blood leaks out into the surrounding brain tissue. If the bleeding continues, the outlook for the future is very poor, with a high risk of dying. However, you have obviously got over this rather dangerous phase and the bleeding has stopped. Your chances of making a good recovery are rather better than those for a similar sized area of dead tissue (infarct). Your doctor will want to try to find a reason for the haemorrhage. High blood pressure, particularly if it has developed only recently, is the most common cause but there are others that might require more investigation.

My son, who is 41, has been taken into hospital with a subarachnoid haemorrhage. What is it all about?

About one in twenty strokes is due to a subarachnoid haemorrhage, which means that there has been bleeding under the membrane that covers the surface of the brain. It is usually due to a weakness in the wall of one of the arteries, called an *aneurysm*, that 'balloons' and then bursts, allowing the blood to escape. It is one of the causes of stroke in young people. Typically it causes a very sudden, severe headache – like being hit hard on the back of the head – followed by stiffness of the neck and an aversion to bright light. There may also be more typical features of stroke, such as paralysis or loss of speech, if some of the leaking blood gets into the brain.

The treatment is different from that for other types of stroke, as an operation may be necessary to repair the aneurysm, so that it doesn't bleed again.

I've been told that I've had an infarction. What is it?

An 'infarction' is the medical term given to an area of tissue that has been damaged as a result of being deprived of its blood supply. The most common cause of this is a blood clot that forms inside one of the arteries and blocks the flow of blood. Infarction is by far the most common form of stroke. They vary in size from just a few millimetres across to those affecting half the brain.

It says in my brother's notes that he has had a CVA. What does that mean?

'CVA' is the abbreviation for 'cerebro-vascular accident'. The term is widely used but is not a good one: many strokes do not affect the cerebrum and none of them is an accident! 'Stroke' is a better term.

I've been told that the investigations show that my stroke was due to an AVM. What is an AVM?

The abbreviation 'AVM' stands for 'arterio-venous malformation'. This is where the structure of the arteries and veins is abnormal. Normally, an artery carrying blood away from the heart branches into lots of smaller arteries and then still smaller blood vessels called capillaries. These capillaries are so narrow that they allow the passage of only one red blood cell at a time. Their walls are very thin and so allow easy transport across of the oxygen and nutrients needed for the cells next to them. The capillaries then join together to form the veins, to return the blood to the heart.

An AVM doesn't have this ordered arrangement: there is a

complex tangle of vessels, the arteries often being directly connected to the veins. These blood vessels are more fragile than normal and can rupture, to cause bleeding into the brain. They are a rare cause of haemorrhage over all, and are usually seen in younger people with stroke. AVMs are generally present from birth, and one doesn't usually know that they are there until they bleed. They can also sometimes cause epileptic fits. If they are found then, it is sometimes desirable to have an operation to remove them before complications develop. If you make a good recovery from your stroke, your doctors will probably want you to have an operation to remove the AVM so that it doesn't bleed again.

My doctor has told me that my brain scan shows that I have had a stroke before, but I don't know anything about it.

Sometimes it is possible to have what is called a silent stroke. Here, part of the brain has been affected that doesn't seem to be doing very much and so there are few, if any, symptoms. They are discovered only when a brain scan is done for some other reason. They are commonly seen, particularly in older people who are having brain scans for some unrelated reason.

Are all strokes the same?

The causes of stroke are many and various. Every individual is different and therefore no one stroke is ever the same as another. The pattern of recovery is different, too. This is what makes it so difficult to predict what is going to happen. Always treat with caution any advice given that seems to be very definite. I [AR] have lost count of the number of times I've been told that 'he was only given a few days to live, and look at him now some years later'. Predictions are particularly difficult to make in the first few weeks after a stroke. As time passes, however, it should be possible for a stroke specialist to make a fairly reasonable estimate of the longer term outlook.

Where has the blood clot that caused my stroke come from?

Blood is more likely to form a clot if its normal smooth flow is disturbed and becomes turbulent – rather like the water in a river when it hits rocks. This can happen in the heart if its rhythm becomes irregular in a condition called *atrial fibrillation,* or in the aorta (the main artery from the heart) or the carotid or vertebral arteries if they become narrowed due to *atheroma* (a build-up of cholesterol in the wall of the artery) – see Figure 5. If a blood clot forms in any of these places, it can either block the artery where it has formed or break off and travel up with the blood to the brain (*embolism*). The clot comes to rest where the artery becomes narrower than the clot, thus preventing any blood getting past it. Sometimes the clot forms in one of the arteries inside the brain itself.

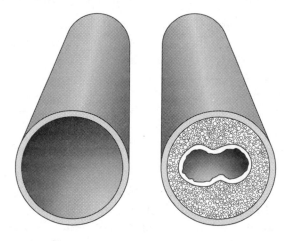

Figure 5 Build-up of atheroma in the arteries gradually blocks the flow of blood

How long will it take for the blood clot to disappear? Where does it go?

Two sorts of blood clot are involved in stroke. The one that has formed inside an artery and is blocking the flow of blood to part of the brain, causing it to be damaged due to lack of oxygen and nourishment, will usually be cleared gradually within a few days or weeks. Blood cells break up the clot and destroy it. Unfortunately, by then the damage will have been done and even if flow in the artery is restored it won't help much. So it doesn't really affect your recovery whether the clot disappears or not.

The second sort of blood clot forms when the wall of an artery bursts inside the brain, allowing blood to leak out around the artery (a cerebral haemorrhage). The blood clot squashes the brain around it, causing damage. In this case, too, the blood clot clears within a few weeks, in much the same way as a bruise elsewhere in your body disappears. As the clot gets smaller, it allows the brain to re-expand into the space previously occupied by the clot and this may allow some of the brain to recover its functions.

Getting better

What is happening to my brain that enables me to recover?

The truthful answer is that we don't really know, but there is a huge amount of research going on to try to understand exactly what happens after a stroke.

When an artery is blocked, the part of the brain it supplies with oxygen and nourishment is affected. There is, however, some overlap between the areas supplied by the arteries, so some of the brain that previously received blood from the blocked artery may still survive, albeit with less blood. There is probably a central portion of brain that depends totally on the blocked artery, and that tissue dies within a few hours. As you move further away from the central damaged area, though, the brain becomes healthier and more likely to survive.

The partially damaged brain may become swollen and inflamed in the same way as the area around a cut does on your finger. Recovery may occur partly as a result of the inflammation settling down and allowing the brain cells to start working again. It may also be due to cells in the area of brain still receiving a little blood 'waking up' and resuming normal activity and to other parts of the brain taking over the functions of the damaged areas of your brain. Although brain cells cannot regenerate once damaged, we do know that the surviving cells can sprout new connections with each other, thus allowing new nerve pathways to develop and function to return. This process is called *neuroplasticity*. There is considerable debate as to how important this is and whether treatment such as physiotherapy may work by encouraging neuroplasticity.

I'm usually quite active, and hate being stuck in bed. How long will it be before I'm back to normal?

This depends on how the stroke affected you. About half to a third of people who have had a stroke will return to normal or nearly normal. The remainder of the survivors will be left with some degree of disability. The pattern of recovery is enormously variable. Some people recover fully within a day or two, while others may have a long hard struggle over many months (some continuing to make improvements two years after their stroke). What determines the speed of recovery is not really clear. It depends, of course, on the severity of the stroke, but that is not the only factor. Your determination to recover is probably very important.

It is usual for the recovery to be fastest at the beginning and then to slow down, although there are people who make little or no recovery for a few weeks and then all of a sudden things start happening. Perhaps to begin with there will be just a flicker of movement at your hip, then your knee and then your arm. Remain optimistic. But always remember that, even if it doesn't all come back, there are ways round difficult problems and life can be very rewarding although there are some things that you can't do as well as you used to.

I want to keep track of my progress. What is the pattern of my recovery going to be?

This is one of the most frequently asked questions and one of the most difficult to answer. The most common pattern is for there to be a few days when not much seems to happen, followed by recovery that happens fastest in the early weeks and then tails off. Recovery in function can still occur at least two years after the stroke. For reasons that we don't fully understand, some functions return faster than others. Often the movement in the leg recovers before the arm, with the hand being the slowest. Loss of sensation is often slower to recover than movement. Neglect or loss of awareness of part of the body (see Chapter 8) is also frequently slow to disappear. Difficulty with swallowing improves in most people within a month. Speech is often one of the slowest aspects to start to recover, but then will continue to get better after everything else has stopped improving.

The nurse told me that my husband has a chest infection but his leg seems weaker and I'm worried he has also had another stroke.

It is very common for a stroke to seem to get worse if other problems, such as a chest infection, develop. While it is of course possible that the stroke has got worse (*extended*), it is likely that the nurse is right and that treating the chest infection will result in the weakness improving to its original level. It is also common for the symptoms of stroke to vary a bit from day to day even without the presence of infection. Don't get dispirited if the recovery doesn't follow an absolutely smooth course. Recovering from a stroke is a bit like climbing a mountain: there are always some down bits on the way up!

My husband has had a stroke before. Does this mean that he won't get better from this one?

The fact that your husband has had a stroke before doesn't mean that his outlook is any worse than after the first one. The amount of his recovery depends on how much damage has been done to his brain. If after the first stroke he was left with a lot of disability, it may be more difficult for him to get going again, both physically and psychologically. On the other hand, he will be an experienced patient and will have learnt a lot of tricks of the trade. A lot depends on his personality and motivation, and the support that you are able to give him.

How much of my daughter's brain has been damaged?

The best way of answering this question is to look at the brain scan. Ask the doctor to explain it to you. Scans are quite easy to understand and will help you to grasp what has happened. On its own, though, a scan is not all that important. Sometimes quite small strokes on the scan can have major effects if they happen in a really important part of the brain, whereas quite large strokes can sometimes produce little noticeable damage. Recovery can be dramatic even if the scan looks horrible.

Can you tell from my CT scan what is going to happen?

The CT scan can only act as a guide. There are many other factors, apart from what parts of your brain have been affected

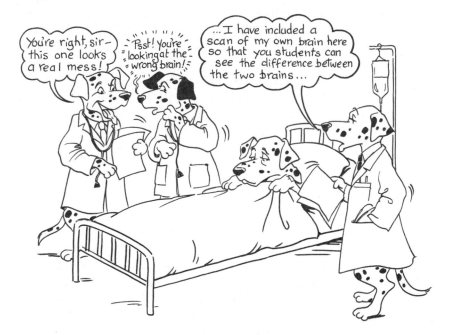

by the stroke, that will determine the speed and extent of your recovery. The scan will help the doctor to decide what the underlying cause might be and whether further investigations are needed, and will also guide treatment and advice about how to prevent another stroke.

Can I ask to see my brain scan?

Yes. Seeing the scan will make it a lot easier for you to understand what is happening.

My husband is completely paralysed down the left side. Does this mean that he is never going to walk again?

No. Even though he may at first have no movement down one side, this does not mean that he can't make a good recovery. The process is a bit like learning to walk as a child. The first stage is for him to regain his balance when sitting. From there the physiotherapist will start getting him to regain his balance when standing and then begin to work on using the strength that will most likely begin to appear in his hip and thigh muscles. It is often a slow and laborious process. Even if your husband doesn't recover full function, he may well be able to walk – perhaps with a stick or frame. At first, walking on a flat hard surface will be the easiest. He will then need to practise on carpet. It often takes a lot of courage to walk outside, partly because the surfaces may be uneven and there is nothing to hold on to and partly because he may feel very self-conscious in public.

My father seems to vary from one day to the next. Sometimes he's awake and alert and other times he's drowsy. Is this normal?

In the early days after a stroke there is often a lot of brain swelling. This may increase the pressure in the brain and can lead to drowsiness or coma. It is quite common for this drowsiness to vary from day to day and does not mean that your father is getting worse. The swelling usually settles within a few weeks.

Even if people are not drowsy, they almost always feel very tired and washed out. It is important not to over-tire your father. His brain can continue recovering even when he is asleep. What sometimes happens, though, is that the normal day/night pattern of wakefulness and sleep gets disturbed and he ends up being awake all night and asleep all day. If this happens, it is worth trying to keep him awake during the day for a few days, so that he is tired when the time for bed comes. Very occasionally, it is necessary for the doctor to prescribe a sleeping tablet for a few nights; this will be just to get him back to the normal day/night rhythm.

The last time I had a stroke I recovered in a few days. Why is it taking so long this time?

Every stroke is different and there is no set pattern to recovery. It may be that a different part of your brain has been affected or that more brain has been damaged than last time. Two strokes that look identical on a brain scan sometimes recover at very different rates. Unfortunately, we don't have all the answers but it is very important not to give up and assume that you are not going to recover at all. Some people are just slower than others!

I've been told that the tests I'm having are to confirm whether or not it is a stroke. What else could it be?

In most cases the diagnosis of stroke made by a doctor taking a careful history and doing a thorough examination will be correct. Occasionally, though, there are other conditions that look like stroke (Table 1). If you take medicine for diabetes, a very low blood sugar can result in temporary paralysis. Some migraine sufferers get temporary symptoms that can seem like a stroke. Although rare, brain tumours can cause symptoms a bit like a stroke, and sometimes a blood clot on the surface of the brain (a *subdural haematoma*) can fool doctors. It is important to find out whether any of these conditions is present, as the treatment will differ. For this reason, most people with stroke-like symptoms should have a brain scan.

Table 1 Conditions that can have symptoms similar to stroke

Epilepsy

Blood clot on the surface of the brain (subdural haematoma)

Brain tumour

Abnormal collections of blood vessels (arterio-venous malformations)

Abnormalities of the blood chemistry (e.g. low levels of sodium or glucose in the blood)

Alcohol intoxication

Drug intoxication

Head injury

Brain abscess

Psychological problems

Not getting better?

My wife seems very ill. What are the chances that she will die?

Every stroke is different, so it is difficult to give a specific answer – but most people who have a stroke do not die. Your doctor probably won't be able to give you absolute assurances, because the illness can be unpredictable, but there are some features that will give pointers to how serious your wife's stroke is. If she remains unconscious or very drowsy for more than a few days, the chances of her pulling through are less. Also, if the brain scan shows a very large area of damage, the outlook is not as good as for a small stroke. For some reason we don't understand, if your wife is still incontinent after a week, her chances of recovery are less.

None of these signs is absolute, though. There are many people who have had all these problems and still made a good recovery. Over all, about a quarter of all people who have a stroke die in the first month. Most deaths happen within the first few days, so the more time that passes the greater the chance that your wife will survive.

My grandfather died immediately when he had a stroke but my wife seems to be well on the mend. Why do people die after a stroke?

In the early days after a stroke, death is usually due to the severity of the brain damage. If the stroke has caused essential parts of the brain such as the breathing centres to stop working, the body cannot go on functioning. Sometimes there is a lot of swelling of the brain as a result the stroke; this can cause pressure to build up inside the head, making it even harder for the brain to continue working.

After the first few days, death from the stroke becomes less likely. If the person still has difficulty swallowing or remains very drowsy, they are at risk of developing chest infections such as pneumonia. Although these infections may respond to antibiotics, they don't always and can make the person's condition get worse. The doctors and nurses will also be concerned to try to prevent blood clots forming in the veins of the paralysed leg, as occasionally these can move, block the flow of blood to the lungs (*pulmonary embolism*) and cause death. The most common cause of death in the weeks immediately after a stroke is a heart attack, but the treatment that the person receives to prevent further strokes will also act to reduce this risk.

The doctors have told me the stroke is so severe that they don't think that my mother will pull through. She spends most of the time asleep and doesn't even seem to know that I'm there. Is she suffering?

I [AR] have never met someone who has come round from the situation you describe who has been able to remember anything that has happened during that stage. Although no one can be absolutely sure what is going on inside the brain of someone who has been severely affected by a stroke, I think it is most unlikely that they are aware of what is going on. Pain is rare after a stroke, although people can get uncomfortable from lying in one position too long or from not having their arms and legs moved. If your mother can't cough very well, phlegm might accumulate at the back of her throat, making her breathing noisy, and that might cause her some distress.

You will know your mother better than any of the staff looking after her: if you think she is getting uncomfortable or distressed, tell the nurses because there are plenty of things they can do to ease her discomfort. Don't be shy to speak on her behalf if she can't do it herself.

My wife was severely disabled before the stroke and this is now the last straw. How do I tell the doctors not to treat her?

You must sit down with the doctors and explain your feelings to them. They can make the decision not to give potentially lifesaving treatments, such as antibiotics for a pneumonia or putting a tube into her stomach to feed her, and it may be that such decisions would be appropriate. In the end though, if your wife is going to pull through, there is nothing the doctors could or would want to do to prevent this.

If my husband is going to end up like a vegetable, he wouldn't want to be kept alive. What should I do?

Discuss with the doctors what their view is of the likely outcome. If they think that the chances of significant recovery are very poor and that the best that can be hoped for is severe paralysis and little mental activity, make it clear what his views were about such a situation. Doctors are not obliged to save life at all costs. There are often times when the right thing to do is to provide everything necessary to relieve suffering but not to interfere with nature taking its course.

It is becoming increasingly common for people to make a 'living will' (an advance directive), in which they say what they want done if they are so ill that a good quality of life would be minimal or non-existent. If your husband has made one, even though it is not legally binding, it will help the doctors in what can sometimes be a difficult decision. It is important that the doctors know what he would want. Your own views and those of the rest of the family are important, but should not be allowed to override those of your husband. In the end, the responsibility for taking the medical decisions should rest with the doctor and nurses, having listened to everything the family has to say. They are the only ones in a position to assess objectively the likely risks and benefits of particular treatments.

2

The first few days

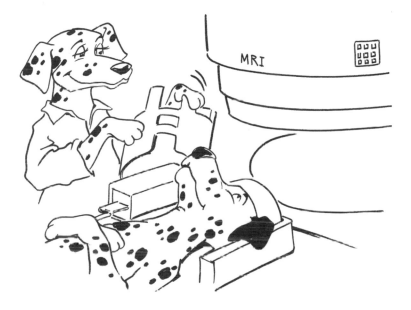

When someone is suspected of having had a stroke, tests will be done to confirm this or to rule it out. Often a brain scan will be done – either CT or MRI.

'CT' is short for *computed tomography*. Introduced in the 1970s, CT scanning revolutionised the investigation of brain disease, because it was now possible to see what was going on inside the brain without difficult, painful and hazardous tests. It has improved enormously, giving much clearer pictures much more quickly. 'MRI' stands for *magnetic resonance imaging*. This method is better than CT scans at showing up very small infarcts, particularly if the doctor thinks the problem is in the cerebellum or the brainstem. The reason for this is that CT scan pictures get distorted, but this is not a difficulty with MRI. The MRI scans can also show up the arteries very clearly (magnetic resonance angiography), and can therefore be used to see where the root of the problem might be.

Other tests may be needed, such as an arteriogram, an echocardiogram or lumbar puncture, and we discuss these too.

The results obtained from the investigations will indicate which treatment is likely to be the best for any particular person. This includes rehabilitation as well as drugs to help recovery.

Investigations

The doctor thinks that I have had a stroke, and is sending me for a brain scan. What will this show?

Nearly everyone who has had a stroke or a suspected stroke should have some sort of brain scan. It helps to confirm the diagnosis and gives more information about the extent and possible underlying cause of the stroke. It is the only reliable way of telling whether the problem is an infarct (an area of dead tissue) or a haemorrhage (bleeding), which is important because the treatment of the two is different. Most stroke specialists think that it is important to do a scan within the first few hours of admission to hospital. The advantage of doing it early is that the doctor can prescribe aspirin with absolute confidence that it won't make matters worse. There is a problem that doing a scan very soon after the onset of the symptoms means there is a strong possibility that it will appear to be normal and won't show the size and exact location of the stroke. This is less of a problem than not knowing as soon as possible whether the stroke is due to a blocked blood vessel (infarct) or a burst blood vessel (haemorrhage). An early scan can nearly always distinguish between these two causes of stroke, so most stroke specialists opt for an early scan, repeating it if necessary.

What is the difference between a CT scan and an MRI scan?

Having a CT scan involves lying on your back, with your head positioned inside the scanner. It takes about five to ten minutes and is completely painless. The doctor may want a scan done after dye is injected into one of your veins, so the injection might be a bit painful. If you are allergic to iodine, make sure the doctor or radiographer knows – in most cases a scan using a dye is not essential.

An MRI scan also involves your lying on your back, and you go into an enclosed tunnel; the machine is quite noisy. (They may play you your favourite music while the scan is being done, to make it slightly more pleasant.) As with a CT scan, it takes only a few minutes, depending on how many bits have to be scanned, and is painless. The MRI machine contains a very powerful magnet, so, if you have any metal bits inside you or a pacemaker, you probably won't be able to have the scan. (It is also very good at wiping clean the magnetic strips on your credit cards!) The tunnel can cause problems for people who get claustrophobic but, because the MRI scan can provide information much more easily than the alternatives, if your doctor advises one, it might be best to grit your teeth and get on with it. If you really think it might be too much, ask if it is possible to have a short-acting sedative to help calm your nerves.

What information does a brain scan give you? Can I ask to see it?

The brain scan will usually tell the medical team the cause and extent of the damage resulting from your stroke. If the doctor doesn't offer to show you your scan, do ask to see it – if you want to. It's your head and it is important that you know as much as possible about what is going on inside it. You are the key person in the rehabilitation process. If you would rather not see it, though, you certainly don't have to.

My wife is to have a carotid doppler. What is it all about?

The carotid doppler is a test that examines the speed of blood flow through the carotid artery. It is completely painless and there is no risk. High-frequency sound waves are produced by a small probe positioned over the neck; the sound waves bounce back when they reach the moving blood, producing a pattern that the radiologist can then look at to determine the blood flow. If your wife's artery is narrowed, the blood flow will be faster; if it is completely blocked, no flow will be detected.

This test is used when there is a suspicion that the stroke might be due to narrowing caused by *atheroma* (build-up of fat) in the carotid artery. This might be suspected if the doctor has heard turbulent flow (a *bruit*) when listening to the artery with a stethoscope. If there is severe narrowing, your wife may be recommended to have an operation to clear the artery (*carotid endarterectomy*).

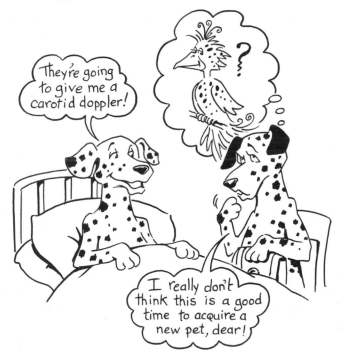

My wife is going to have an arteriogram. What is it, and what is it for?

An arteriogram is an X-ray taken to show the inside of the arteries. It can be done by injecting dye either direct into one of the arteries (usually through the groin) or, more often, into a vein in the arm. This test will often be done if there is concern that there might be an *aneurysm* (a small ballooning of the wall of the artery) that might have leaked, most commonly causing a subarachnoid haemorrhage. It might also be performed after a cerebral haemorrhage to try to see if there are any other abnormalities of the blood's circulation in the brain. If one of these problems is found in your wife, an operation might be recommended to prevent it from happening again.

It is often possible to avoid the need for arteriography by using an MRI scan to show the blood vessels.

They keep taking blood from me. Why do they need so much?

This is one of the most common complaints of people in hospital beds. It isn't because we are vampires! Examining your blood can tell us a great deal about the way your body is working. Even though your brain is the immediate cause of the trouble, it is important to make sure that, for example, your liver and kidneys are healthy. You may well be given drugs after the stroke that need to be monitored to make sure they do not cause any untoward effects. Tests can also be performed on your blood that tell us why you have had a stroke. Make sure you ask your doctors what the blood tests are for and what the results are.

The doctor says I might have to have a trans-oesophageal echocardiogram. What is this, and what is it for?

Just as the blood flow in the carotid arteries can be examined, so the way the heart is working can be studied using a Doppler probe. It can detect whether the valves of the heart are functioning normally, how thick the walls of the chambers of the heart are and whether there is a blood clot present that could have been the cause of the stroke. In most instances this *echocardiogram* is done by moving the probe over the front of the chest overlying the heart.

Sometimes a clearer view is needed of particular bits of the heart, which can only be done by getting a view from behind the heart. This is when the doctor will ask for a *trans-oesophageal echocardiogram*. The back of your throat will be sprayed to make it numb, and you will be asked to swallow the small probe attached to a wire. When it is positioned about half-way down your gullet (oesophagus) the probe will start producing detailed images of your heart. The procedure takes about 10–15 minutes. Although sometimes it is a bit uncomfortable, it is not painful and is not a risky procedure.

My next-door neighbour who had a stroke had a lumbar puncture. Should I have had one?

Only very rarely is it necessary to have a lumbar puncture after stroke. It is sometimes needed to confirm a diagnosis of subarachnoid haemorrhage and occasionally a sample of spinal fluid is required to look for rare causes of stroke. A lumbar puncture should never be done without you first having a brain scan.

If you do have a lumbar puncture, you will be asked to lie on your side. Local anaesthetic is injected to numb the skin of your lower back and the needle inserted into the spinal canal. Fluid is then removed. There is no risk of damaging your spinal cord, because the needle is placed below the lower end of the cord. The main side effect is that some people develop a headache, which can last for a few days afterwards. The headache occurs because the amount of fluid around the brain is slightly lower than normal – just like the headache with a hangover.

I was told I need a swallowing assessment in the X-ray department. What is it?

If there is concern that your normal swallowing reflex has been affected by the stroke, the speech and language therapist – in collaboration with the doctor – may recommend that you have a *video-fluoroscopy*. This involves making a video film of X-rays while you swallow a barium mixture made up into different consistencies. The film will show whether any of the barium is going down the wrong way, into your lungs. It will also help to see precisely what is wrong with your swallowing so that the speech and language therapist can give you the correct advice about the amounts and consistencies it is safe for you to eat and drink.

Some hospitals use a different technique to assess how safe it is to swallow – called *fibreoptic endoscopic evaluation of swallowing* (FEES). This involves the speech therapist passing a flexible tube with a light into the back of your throat through which they can directly observe what happens when you swallow. You may have heard about a similar procedure being done – a *gastroscopy* – to look at the stomach in people who might have ulcers. It uses a similar instrument but, of course, for assessing your swallow doesn't need to be passed all the way down the gullet. It is very easy to do (usually on the ward), safe and not too uncomfortable.

Treatment

A friend was telling me about something called a clot-busting drug. Should I have been treated with this?

In recent years the treatment of people with heart attacks has been dramatically improved by using *thrombolysis* – giving 'clot-busting drugs' such as streptokinase and tissue plasminogen activator (tPA). They work by causing rapid destruction of the blood clot blocking the artery, allowing normal blood flow to resume and preventing permanent damage to the heart muscle. Their successful use in heart disease made us optimistic that there might be similar benefits after stroke. There have been several medical trials, the one receiving the most publicity being performed in the USA using recombinant tissue plasminogen activator (rtPA). Giving the drug within three hours of the first symptoms of stroke resulted in slightly lower death rates and disability when measured three months later. On the basis of this study, the drug has been licensed for use in the USA and is being fairly widely used there. It has only recently been licensed for use in Europe, and in the UK very little is being given. It is likely that it will become more widely available over the next few years as more stroke units are established, and more stroke specialists are appointed.

If it is going to be given, though, we will have to radically change our approach to the early care of people with stroke. The general public will need to become much more aware of the symptoms of stroke and call for medical assistance more quickly, because the drug must be given within three hours of the symptoms starting; the ambulance crews will need to treat stroke with much more urgency; in hospital accident and emergency departments, brain scanning will have to be immediately available because it would be dangerous to give clot-busting drugs to someone with a brain haemorrhage. At present, in many parts of the UK, people are still sitting on hospital trolleys waiting to be seen three hours after their stroke.

The benefits of rtPA are real, but it needs to be given by people who know exactly what they are doing. In the wrong hands it can be an extremely dangerous treatment resulting in greater levels of death and disability. If there was a stroke near a centre that was experienced in giving the drug, I [AR] would opt to have it. Anywhere else, though, I would let nature decide what was going to happen.

Are there any risks associated with thrombolysis?

Yes, there is a risk of bleeding into the brain. This happens in about 5% of people treated with the drug. It can be very serious, in some cases leading to death. The risks can be minimised by the drug being given only by people who are experienced giving it, in a centre that is set up for the purpose. Thrombolysis should not be given by amateurs.

Are there any other drugs I could have been treated with?

The only drug that has clearly been shown to be beneficial after stroke is aspirin and then only for infarcts and not haemorrhage (i.e. for blockages and not for bleeding). There are a lot of new drugs at various stages of development, some of which may make their way onto the market within the next few years. Many of these are in the group of drugs called *neuroprotectors*, which are designed to reduce the amount of damage to the nerve cells in the area around the central core of dead brain tissue. Many drugs are prescribed in other countries around Europe for stroke, usually with extravagant claims for their benefit. There is no justification for using any of these.

I've been put on a special mattress, which makes it difficult to sleep. Why can't I have an ordinary mattress?

If you have difficulty moving in bed after your stroke, it is very important to make sure that you don't develop any pressure sores. They are terribly easy to get, especially if your skin is a bit thin and you are sleepy. Once they develop, they can be extremely uncomfortable and take ages to heal. For these reasons, it is routine for the nurses to check, when you arrive on the ward, whether you are at risk of developing a pressure sore. If they think you are, you will have a special mattress put onto your bed which will relieve the pressure. These mattresses are of varying types, but most involve air cells inflating and deflating every few minutes. Unfortunately, they can be a bit uncomfortable and most are a bit noisy as well. It's a small price to pay for preventing a sore, though, and as soon as you are a bit fitter you'll be back on an ordinary hospital mattress. You might then be pleading for the other one back!

When I had an operation I was told that I had to have heparin injections to prevent me from getting a thrombosis in my leg because I couldn't get out of bed. Shouldn't I have heparin now after my stroke?

The risk of developing a blood clot in the veins of a leg paralysed by a stroke is quite high. Unfortunately, a large trial of giving heparin after stroke showed that, over all, it was more harmful than helpful. The advice usually given, therefore, is to wear anti-thrombosis stockings, get the leg moving as quickly as possible and make sure that you take plenty of fluids so that you don't get dehydrated.

My mother has a drip. Why is this?

A *drip* is a tube inserted into a vein to allow fluids or drugs to be given direct into the blood stream. It is one of those things that get put in without necessarily much thought in the accident and emergency department, and then it stays put. If a drip is in place, it shouldn't be left for more than a few days without being replaced, as it can make the area around it inflamed or infected. This is always a good time to question the necessity of continuing with the drip.

Whether a drip is necessary depends entirely on how well your mother is drinking and if she needs drugs to be given direct into a vein. Everyone should drink at least one and a half litres of liquid a day – possibly more in hospital, where it is often very hot. If your mother is allowed to have 'free' (unlimited) fluids, make sure that she has enough access to drinks that she likes (not alcohol in the first few days at least) and try to encourage her to take plenty. If the drinks need thickening, it is more difficult to keep up with fluid requirements and even greater attention should be paid to making sure that your mother has enough to drink.

Why isn't my partner connected up to some oxygen?

Unless there is definite evidence that his blood oxygen level is low, there is no need for extra oxygen. In fact, being attached to unnecessary tubes may even hinder the rehabilitation process. If, however, the oxygen monitor shows that the oxygen concentration in the blood (*oxygen saturation*) is low, oxygen should be given to try to reduce the amount of brain that eventually dies as a result of the stroke.

If stroke is such a serious illness, shouldn't my husband be in an intensive care unit?

So long as he is in a ward with nurses experienced in managing people with stroke, it is likely that he will be receiving the level of care needed in the early phase of the illness. There are no high-technology treatments or investigations that require the level of care provided in an intensive care unit.

If aspirin helps prevent another stroke, why won't they give my partner this until after she has had a brain scan?

The research trials have clearly shown that there is a small benefit in terms of death rates and level of disability if 300mg of aspirin is begun within 48 hours of the start of symptoms of a stroke caused by lack of blood flow (*ischaemic stroke*). However, giving your partner aspirin could worsen a stroke due to a cerebral haemorrhage. A scan is essential to determine whether the stroke is due to infarct or to haemorrhage (blockage or bleeding).

In fact, many of the people who took part in the aspirin trials were started on the treatment without first having a scan. If there has to be a choice between not having the aspirin because it is not possible to get a scan in time and having it but taking the small risk of making things worse, we would opt for the aspirin. But if we were in the Far East, where haemorrhage is much more common, the balance would swing the other way. Clearly the ideal solution is an early scan and then start appropriate treatment.

If the brain swells up after a stroke, aren't there any treatments that could reduce the swelling?

Unfortunately, none of the drugs that have been tried so far has been successful. Some drugs that have been used, such as steroids, can actually cause harm. There is a technique that involves an operation to remove some of the skull bone so as to relieve the pressure in the underlying brain and this is occasionally used for people with massive brain swelling, especially when the stroke affects the right side of the brain. It has not yet undergone proper clinical trials and so has not yet achieved wide acceptance in the UK.

What side effects will I get from the drugs?

The main drug that you are likely to be treated with in the early stages of your illness is aspirin, which is a very safe drug when taken in the very low doses that are given for stroke. Aspirin has to be used with caution in people with a history of stomach ulcers, as it can cause irritation, and bleeding, of the lining of the stomach. If this is a problem, there are three options:

- add a drug to protect the stomach (e.g. ranitidine or cimetidine),

- use an alternative to aspirin (e.g. dipyridamole or clopidogrel),

- not give anything at all.

Unless the bleeding has been within the last couple of years, doctors will often try aspirin with a stomach-protecting drug. Occasionally, people are allergic to aspirin, developing a rash or having difficulty with breathing if they take any. If this is the case, aspirin should definitely not be used.

The only other drugs commonly used in the early stages after stroke are laxatives (for constipation) or pain-killers, neither of which is likely to cause much in the way of problems.

I have read that cooling people down might help save brain tissue. Is this true?

We have known for many years that cooling the body can reduce its oxygen requirements, and this procedure is now routine during complex heart surgery, giving the surgeon longer to operate. In experimental studies, cooling animals after causing a stroke results in significantly less brain injury than if the animal is kept at normal temperature. Experiments of cooling after stroke have not yet been done in people, but they probably will be within the next few years and it wouldn't be surprising if ten years from now it was a routine part of stroke care. Already there is a centre in Germany that is lowering the body temperature to 32°Celsius (89.6°Fahrenheit) for very severe stroke. The initial reports are encouraging but need to be tested in a formal trial first, before it can be recommended.

Other evidence that suggests controlling temperature might be important is the observation that people who develop a fever after a stroke do less well than those who maintain a normal temperature. Whether this is because people with a more severe stroke are more likely to develop a high temperature or that the fever itself is harmful to a brain that has recently sustained a stroke is not clear. Research is needed to see if it is helpful to give paracetamol to people with fever, to bring down their temperature after a stroke.

Would an operation help to remove the blood clot?

There are a few circumstances where an operation after a stroke is helpful, but only a few. The major one is where there is a large bleed into the part of the brain called the cerebellum. A blood clot here might cause a big rise in the pressure within the head, which can be very dangerous. Removing the clot from this area has been helpful in preventing this rise in pressure, with an overall improved outcome. Occasionally, strokes elsewhere in the brain can cause a rise in pressure (hydrocephalus) and an operation to remove the clot or to put in a *shunt* (a device to drain excess fluid away from the brain) might be needed.

There is little evidence so far that operating to remove clots from elsewhere in the brain is better than leaving nature to remove them, although surgery is often the preferred treatment ('treatment of choice') outside the UK.

Although clots in the arteries are the cause of most strokes, there are no useful operations to remove them from the arteries.

My husband has had a subarachnoid haemorrhage. What is his treatment likely to be?

Subarachnoid haemorrhage – bleeding onto the surface of the brain – is managed very differently from other sorts of stroke. Often people are looked after in neuro-surgical units rather than in medical wards, because there is a much greater chance that surgery will eventually be needed. The worry with subarachnoid haemorrhage is that bleeding might recur. The time when this is most likely is in the first three weeks after the initial bleed, so it is usual to try to find the cause of the haemorrhage. If an aneurysm (a weak spot in an artery) is found, an operation to repair it will be done as soon as possible. It is also particularly important to keep careful control of the blood pressure to make sure it doesn't rise too high. A drug called nimodipine is often given to reduce the spasm in the damaged vessels, which may also help prevent further brain damage due an inadequate blood supply.

There can also be problems as with other types of cerebral haemorrhage, such as paralysis, difficulty with swallowing, difficulty with speech and so on. All the aspects of rehabilitation discussed in the next section, 'Rehabilitation issues', therefore apply, too.

Is there any treatment available that I could pay for that might help me?

Treatments that are not often available on the NHS but that might help include acupuncture, massage, aromatherapy and most of the other forms of 'complementary medicine'. There is some research evidence to support the use of acupuncture but otherwise these treatments have not been proven to be of any use. On the other hand, they haven't been shown to be harmful and they can be very pleasant.

We are not aware of any worthwhile conventional medicine that you can't get on the NHS – with the possible exception of Viagra. There are certainly no other drugs that, if you pay for them privately, will have any magical effects.

I'm confused by all the different people working on the ward. What do they all do?

Running an effective hospital takes a huge number of staff, many of whom you probably never see, such as those working in the kitchens, those preparing sterile equipment, the technical staff, personnel and so on.

On the ward, most staff will be the nurses. They will have varying degrees of seniority, currently graded from A (untrained junior nursing assistants) to G or H (ward managers). Qualified nurses (Registered General Nurses, RGNs) will be from grade D upwards. It is likely that the nurses' uniforms will vary according to their seniority. There will be some ward domestics, who help to keep the ward clean and tidy and help out with serving meals and drinks.

The therapists may have responsibilities on more than one ward. It is very likely that you will have contact with a physiotherapist, an occupational therapist and, possibly, a speech and language therapist. There may also be a psychologist, although they are few and far between. There will probably be a dietitian, who will be there to give advice if there are particular issues about your nutrition. The pharmacist will be there to check your drug charts to make sure the doctors haven't made any mistakes, to make sure the ward has enough stock of the prescribed medicines and to tell you about the medicines they will give you to take home with you.

The number of doctors will vary. Your care will almost certainly be supervised by a consultant. He or she will have been qualified as a doctor for at least ten years and will have been trained in one speciality for the final few of these years. Those most commonly responsible for the care of people with strokes are physicians for the elderly, neurologists (specialists in conditions affecting the brain, nerves and muscles) and general physicians. There are now a small number of physicians whose primary role is caring for stroke patients, and it is likely that their number will increase in the next few years. Being supervised by the consultant will probably be a middle grade doctor such as a specialist registrar or an associate specialist, and a junior doctor at junior or senior house officer level. You will see most of the junior doctors. Their responsibilities will be to check on you most days, keep abreast of what is happening to you and report back to their seniors on the ward rounds. In addition to all these staff, you will also be aware of the people who come and keep taking blood off you (the phlebotomists). The porters are vital in maintaining the smooth running of the hospital, particularly in large hospitals where you might spend a large proportion of your time being wheeled from one end to the other!

Hopefully, all the staff will be wearing name badges. If they aren't or you don't know what someone does, do ask.

Rehabilitation issues

How soon should I be starting rehabilitation? What can be done immediately?

Rehabilitation should start immediately the stroke happens. It is not a process that begins when the admitting doctor gets bored and decides the time has come to move you on to a rehabilitation unit! Not paying attention to aspects of rehabilitation from the outset can cause problems that might take a long time to resolve. For example, if you have a paralysed arm, it is very easy to end up with a painful shoulder because the arm has been positioned incorrectly or someone has pulled on the arm while trying to lift you. Being left lying in bed for long periods, without any effort to get you to sit up, might delay the return of your balance when sitting. It could make it more likely that you get blood clots in your legs or pressure sores, and you might find it more difficult to swallow enough liquids and food to keep you healthy. There are many aspects to the process of rehabilitation after a stroke, physical and psychological. Clearly, it is vital to get the diagnosis right and give you the correct medicines, but it is equally important to work on getting you to regain your normal functions.

What needs to be done immediately depends a lot on what problems you have. If there is any significant paralysis, it is important to begin concentrating on your balance, first in bed and then sitting in a chair. Making sure that your arms and legs are always positioned correctly and putting them through the full range of movement so that they don't get stiff or painful will prevent delays later in your treatment.

Paying careful attention to your swallowing, nutrition and fluid intake is critical; you may not be in the best position to decide for yourself what is really necessary. It is also important that you understand exactly what is being done and what is expected of you. If staff sometimes forget to give you full information, do ask what is happening. Knowing what is going on, and why, should go a long way to preventing a perfectly natural feeling of helplessness and depression. Moreover, your treatment should not make you more disabled than you already are! For example, people often have a urinary catheter inserted on their arrival at the hospital, without a good reason, but how can you be expected to keep your bladder working properly with a rubber tube continually draining your urine? If you can just about walk five metres, why position your bed ten metres from the nearest toilet? If you can get out of bed with a bit of a struggle, try doing it independently with the cot sides up! For every individual with a stroke there is a different list of things that need to be done. There always is a long list, so don't put up with nothing being done.

I don't want to go into hospital. Can I be treated at home?

The answer depends to some extent on how severe your stroke was and the access you would have to medical and nursing help. Anything is possible given the right resources, but it is likely to be more difficult to provide the appropriate level of care at home. Many of the tests – such as the scans – can only be done at the hospital, and travelling backwards and forwards may not be easy or desirable for you. If you have any difficulty eating or drinking properly and you require a drip or feeding tube, it becomes very difficult to get this sort of care at home. You may well require nursing care 24 hours a day to prevent, for example, pressure sores. Unless you are paying privately, it is unlikely that the health and social services will have sufficient resources to provide the necessary care day and night. Even relatively simple increases in the amount of personal care you might need could be difficult to organise quickly enough to cover the important early few days after your stroke.

If your stroke was very mild, it is feasible to consider remaining at home. Nevertheless, a few days in hospital to get a specialist opinion and have all the important tests done is a sensible way to proceed.

Once you are over the initial phase of your illness, specialist rehabilitation at home is probably as effective as specialist rehabilitation in hospital. What is not acceptable, however, is simply being discharged early to an inadequate community rehabilitation programme being provided by non-specialists. Services vary from area to area and you will need to ask the team looking after you, or your GP, what is available and what the reasonable options are for you. It is very important not to compromise the quality of your care in the early weeks after a stroke just because, for example, you dislike hospitals.

My wife is in a stroke unit. How is this different from other hospital wards?

Stroke units are wards that specialise in treating people who have had a stroke. A lot of research has been conducted into the value of stroke units and the evidence is clear: people looked after in a stroke unit do better after their stroke than people cared for in a general medical or geriatric ward. Precisely what it is about stroke units that is better is not absolutely certain, but there are a few key differences in the way that care is provided.

- The nursing staff have far greater experience of helping to rehabilitate people after their strokes.

- The therapists spend about an hour or so with each patient a day. For the other 23 hours, if any therapy is to be given it will be up to the nurses and visitors.

- All staff, both qualified and unqualified, will have had training about stroke and therefore will have greater expertise.

- They will be working as a multi-professional team, co-ordinating their efforts to get their patients better. It is usual for such a team to include doctors, nurses, physiotherapists, occupational therapists, speech and language therapists, social workers and sometimes psychologists, pharmacists and dietitians.

- The team will involve your wife and her carers (such as you) in the whole process of rehabilitation, so that everyone is working to agreed targets.

- The stroke unit will have built up close links with all the services available in the community that might be needed after discharge. In this way returning home should be easier for your wife.

I'm longing to get home to my own bed! How long will I have to be in hospital?

In Britain the average length of stay in hospital after a stroke is 35 days. Of course, with milder strokes it is shorter than for more severe cases. Other factors that will determine how long you will need to stay include:

- What is your home like? For example, will you have to climb stairs?

- What are the services like in your area for continuing rehabilitation after you are discharged?

- How much support will you have from friends and relatives at home?

- What are your preferences for treatment?

It is important to realise that the initial period of care in hospital is just the first stage in the rehabilitation process and that not everything will, or indeed can, be achieved by the time you go home. Only when you are back, attempting to resume your normal routines, will you truly find out what you still need to work on. A lot of the psychological adjustment that may be needed can only really be achieved when you are back home. The staff on the ward should discuss your progress with you throughout your stay, so that when you are discharged it won't be a surprise and you will be both physically and psychologically prepared for it.

I'm not being treated on a stroke unit – I don't think my hospital has one. What should I do?

In a recent study of the management of stroke in the UK, only 27% of people spent more than half of their stay in a stroke unit, although about 75% of hospitals had one. Clearly, therefore, there is a long way to go to achieve universally good quality care. There are a lot more stroke units now than there were ten years ago and hospital trusts are beginning to get the message that stroke units are worth investing in. Probably one of the best ways of persuading trusts to change is for patients and their representatives to complain about the service that is being provided. A letter to the chief executive will often produce more action more quickly than any request from a consultant or manager. Although it won't help you this time, you will be helping to change things for the future.

Something else you can do is learn as much as possible about stroke and how it should be treated, and try to demand that you get treated in that way even if you are not in a stroke unit. It is unfortunate but true that knowledgeable demanding people get more than the passive uncomplaining ones.

It is difficult to get transferred from one hospital to another so as to get into a stroke unit. It is likely that the nearest stroke unit will be full, treating its own local residents, and most such units have a policy of not accepting transfers from out of their area without a very good reason. You can, of course, always try. You never get anything you don't ask for!

There are, however, negative aspects to being moved away from your local hospital. It will be further for visitors to get to, and when you are discharged it may be more difficult to organise services from a hospital some distance away from your home.

Although my hospital doesn't have a stroke unit, it does have a rehabilitation ward. Is that all right?

It is less important what a unit is called than what the staff are like. Committed nurses, therapists and doctors with experience in rehabilitation are essential. Stroke accounts for about half of the rehabilitation that hospitals need to provide, so it is very likely that a general rehabilitation ward will have considerable experience of looking after people such as you. Certainly if the choice is between a general ward and a rehabilitation ward, we would choose the rehabilitation ward. Find out as much as possible about the sort of treatment you need and then discuss with the staff on the unit how they are going to help you get it.

The stroke unit is full of old people and I feel out of place. What can I do?

This is a common feeling when people first arrive in a stroke unit. The fact is that about half of all strokes happen to people over the age of 75 years and three-quarters in people over 65. Stroke is therefore quite uncommon in younger people, although it can and does happen to people of all ages, including children. Although there are special problems that need to be addressed in the rehabilitation of younger people with strokes, most of the issues are identical whatever your age. It is more important that you are looked after by professionals who know how best to treat you than being in a ward with younger people but being looked after by people with little knowledge or interest in your condition. So our advice is to put up with it. In fact, of course, old people are not really much different from young ones. Certainly they often suffer from more illness and probably have more wrinkles than you, but otherwise they are as varied and as likeable, or not, as people of any generation.

The nurses don't seem as helpful as they were on the other ward. They are always telling me to do things myself and it's really difficult.

The role of nursing staff in stroke units and rehabilitation units is rather different from that of general nurses. They are there to help you get back to being independent, which won't happen if they do everything for you. If you have ever had children or worked in teaching, you will know that it is often easier to do the job yourself rather than making someone do it for themselves. But if they are ever going to learn, you have to be patient and encouraging. That is what your nurses are probably doing when they tell you to try to do it yourself. If you really can't do it, tell them and then they will show you how it can be done or they will do it for you.

Having said all that, there may be occasions when you come across a rude or lazy member of staff who really can't be bothered. People like this exist in every organisation, and nurses are not always angels. If you are unfortunate enough to be faced with one of these, talk to the ward manager. They will view your concerns seriously and take appropriate action.

The nurses always get my wife out of bed using a hoist rather than lifting her. She doesn't like the hoist. It's uncomfortable and she gets frightened. Why won't they lift her?

Too many nurses are still injured every year lifting people. There are now European Union directives that dictate how much weight a nurse may lift, and this may be why your wife is being transferred in a hoist. It is undignified and can be a bit frightening at first, but usually the hoist is only needed in the early stages after the stroke; as soon as she is able to take a bit of weight on her legs, the nurses will be able to transfer her with one or two people instead of the hoist. In the meantime, it could be worth mentioning your wife's fears to the nurses, as they might have alternative slings that they could try with the hoist – this will give her greater support and make her feel less insecure.

I'm frightened that my wife is going to fall out of bed. I have asked the nurses to put up cot sides but they've refused, saying it's not hospital policy.

Cot sides are needed only very occasionally and, far from preventing injuries, can actually cause harm. They tend to be used when people are restless in bed and there is a fear that they will fall. In these circumstances I [AR] have seen the restlessness made worse as the person in bed struggles to get free from a restraint that they don't understand. It is easy to trap an arm between the bars and then break it, and occasionally people have managed to get over the side of the bars and fall from an even greater height to the floor than they would have done without the bars.

The other problem with cot sides is that they severely limit rehabilitation. It is completely the wrong message to give to the person who has had the stroke, their carers and the staff – the patient has to be restrained behind bars. There are two ways to wind up behind bars: one is to commit a crime and end up in prison, and the other is to fall ill and end up in hospital. At least the criminal knows how long his sentence is!

There is, unfortunately, no way to have an effective rehabilitation programme without some risks being taken. If the staff do everything in their power to keep your wife safe from falls, she will be less likely to be able to walk again or be independent in other activities. If you are worried that your wife will fall out of bed because she is restless, a better solution than cot sides is for the mattress to be put directly on the floor. If she always tends to roll in one particular direction, putting that side of the bed against the wall might reduce the risk. Placing crash mats round the side of the bed will reduce the likelihood of her hurting herself.

Identifying what is making her restless might be the key to preventing a fall:

- Is she in pain?

- Is the bed uncomfortable?

- Is she too hot or cold?

- Is she getting cramps in her paralysed leg?

Experiment to find out what makes her most comfortable. Discuss with the nurses whether they feel that her bed is best placed for them to be able to keep a close eye on your wife, particularly at night. It might be worth moving her out of the single room and onto the main ward near the nurses' desk. There are instances when it is appropriate to use cot sides – but only when all the other options have been tried or at least considered, and then only for as short a time as possible.

My wife had a fall when she was in the rehabilitation unit. Surely something should have been done to prevent it?

Precautions can be taken to prevent falls but we would be very worried to hear that a rehabilitation unit never has any falls. This would mean that they are being too protective of the people they are trying to rehabilitate, and are probably not doing their job properly. In the answer to the previous question are listed some of the things that can be done to prevent falls or injuries from falls. But in the end the only way to be absolutely sure that your wife never falls again is to tie her into her chair and bed with strong straps. Not advisable!

I would much prefer to be in a single room but have been advised that I'm better in the main ward. Why is this?

There are some good reasons why being in a single room is not always ideal. It is difficult for the nursing staff to be as aware of what is happening to you as they would be if you were more visible on the main ward. Even if the nurses are not around, sharing a bay with three or four other people means that they may be able to help or call for help if you need it. Rehabilitation after a stroke is about stimulating the brain, getting it to wake up and form new connections between the healthy brain cells. So it is important for you to be surrounded as much as possible by sights and sounds and even smells. It may be irritating and noisy at times when you want to rest, but it is probably better for you to be in that sort of environment than being left with only your thoughts to stimulate your brain.

The price that you pay is loss of some privacy. With only a curtain between you and the next bed it is difficult to keep many secrets. All rooms on wards now need to be single sex, unless there is some dire emergency. Good quality nursing should be able to maintain some privacy. If you want to have private conversations with your visitors or a member of staff, there will be a room somewhere nearby that you could go to. If you can't walk, ask to borrow a wheelchair and get yourself pushed off the ward to somewhere that you can talk without being disturbed. The ward is not a prison and there is usually no good reason why you should not be allowed to leave it for a while.

There are times when being looked after in a single room is a good idea. If one of the patients is very noisy, it makes sense to put them on their own. Single rooms are desirable when young mothers have to be in hospital. A single room is also used for nursing someone who is very sick and needs a lot of attention, and when friends and family need privacy to be with them. It can be very useful towards the end of your stay in hospital. If you are going home to live on your own and there are some concerns about how you will cope, letting you try it out in a room set up to be a little like your own home can help identify what the problems might be and work out the solutions. Most NHS hospitals have only a few single rooms, which have to be used in the most appropriate way. In the end it is the ward manager's decision but, if you are keen to get one, you should ask.

I spend so much time sitting on the ward doing nothing. Surely I would get out of here more quickly if I was worked harder?

It is now generally agreed that more intensive rehabilitation gets better results, so sitting around doing nothing for most of the day is unhelpful. Discuss with your therapists what your programme is for the week: find out from them and the nursing staff what objectives have been set for you and what you can do to achieve them. Although it is likely that the physiotherapist, occupational therapist and speech therapist will be able to give you only perhaps half an hour each of individual therapy a day, there may be 'homework' that can be set. Getting your visitors involved can also be helpful, and will give them something else to do other than eat your grapes and read your magazines.

Much of the therapy after a stroke is centred around normal activities of daily living. For example, getting washed and dressed in the morning involves a very complex series of physical and intellectual processes that may need to be learnt again after a stroke. The nurses should be encouraging you to do as much of such tasks as possible for yourself – this is all part of rehabilitation. Throughout the day there are things happening to you that are opportunities for rehabilitation. So don't think that the only therapy you get is when you are in the gym.

Particularly in the early stages of recovery, it is possible to do too much therapy. You will need more rest and sleep than you are used to and you should take advice from the staff as to what level of activity is in your best interests. The type of activity that you do is also important. It is possible to cause harm by doing the wrong things, so again take advice from the experts.

Would I get better care if I went privately?

There is very little specialist stroke rehabilitation available privately in the UK. In most cases the care that the NHS provides is excellent but there may be instances where it falls short of the ideal, in which case it might be worth considering private care. It is, though, likely to be very costly. Many of the private insurance companies refuse to pay for the rehabilitation phase of treatment after a stroke, and there have been many instances where people have been discharged from a private hospital too early. If you are funding yourself, there may be several months of care to pay for at many hundreds of pounds a day. It is probably worth keeping your money and using it to pay for some extra therapy when you are back home or for a holiday in the sun when you are a bit better. Having something to look forward to is very important and really will help pull you through what may be some very grey days in hospital.

I'd really like to go home. Is it absolutely necessary to be in hospital to have rehabilitation?

No. Once you are over the phase of your illness that requires intensive treatment in hospital – such as drips, drugs being given directly into veins, oxygen and so on – care can be provided at home just as well as in hospital. The important thing is for the rehabilitation to be provided by a specialist stroke team. If such a team is available only in your hospital, it will be better for you to stay there. If there is a community team, though, there is no reason not to use it so long as your home environment is appropriate.

All the other people in my unit are much older than me. Are there any special units in the UK for young people who have had a stroke?

There are very few if any specialist stroke units specifically for younger people, although there are several general rehabilitation centres that concentrate on people under 65 years of age. If you feel very strongly, it might be worth discussing with your doctors whether it is possible to transfer to one of these. But do first consider the possible disadvantages:

- It is likely that the unit will be a long way from home and will be difficult for visitors to get to.

- When it comes to planning your discharge, the unit will not

necessarily know very much about the services that are
available in your area.

- Although you may be surrounded by younger people in the
  new unit, they might have needs very different from yours.

- Many of the specialist rehabilitation units for young people
  have long waiting lists or take a long time to get into
  because of cumbersome assessment procedures. By the
  time you get there, will you still need in-patient treatment?

On the plus side, however, they may be much better set up to
help you solve problems such as getting back the skills you need
to return to work. Your doctor or therapist will know or be able
to find out what your options are, so discuss it with them.

3
Getting moving again

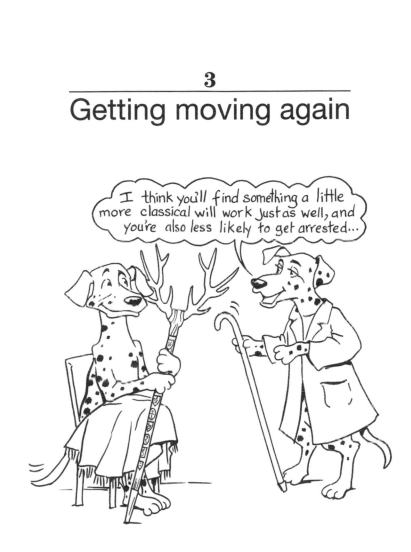

One of the most important aspects of your treatment will be to get you moving again. The two specialists who will be helping you with this will be the physiotherapist and the occupational therapist, but the other staff will be involved too. Your family and friends can also help if they have been shown what to do.

Physiotherapy

What part will the physiotherapist play in helping me to get better?

The physiotherapist will be helping you to regain as much muscle function as possible and then to use that function to regain normal movement. If full muscle strength is not likely to return, the physiotherapist will help in getting you to function to the best of your ability, perhaps with the aid of a stick or some other piece of equipment.

The physiotherapist will become involved in your care very soon after the stroke, unless you have absolutely no problems with movement. If you are still at the stage of being in bed and wholly dependent on the nurses, you will need the physiotherapist's advice as to the best positions in which to lie. Your limbs will need to be moved for you (passive movement) if you can't do it yourself, to prevent the muscles and joints from getting too stiff. As soon as you are awake enough, you will be sat out in a chair. To begin with it is likely that you will find it difficult staying upright, and the physiotherapist will be working with you to help you regain normal balance. One of the common difficulties after a stroke is that people lose their sense of where their 'midline' (the imaginary line that divides the body into left and right sides) is. As a result, they may think they are sitting up straight when they are actually leaning over to one side. Depending on your particular problems, the physiotherapist may then move on to getting you standing with the support of a hoist or two or three people. This will encourage you to use the muscles in your trunk and, hopefully, around your hips (pelvis). It will also help your balance.

Recovery of muscle function usually begins in the back and around the buttocks. The leg usually starts moving before the arm. The physiotherapist will be following this natural pattern of recovery, making sure that you are using your muscles in as normal a way as possible.

I'm about to start physiotherapy. How often should I be having it?

This of course depends on the severity of your stroke and the stage you are at in recovery. If you still need to be in hospital and have problems with movement, it would be reasonable to expect to have a session of physiotherapy daily on weekdays, lasting between half an hour and one hour. The length of the therapy session will depend on how much you can tolerate as much as on how much time the therapist has available, though having an extra few minutes of therapy a day in addition to what is usually provided does produce a little extra benefit. Later on in the course of your recovery it may well be possible to reduce the frequency of the therapy sessions to perhaps two or three a week, with you doing the exercises in between.

Is it important that I get treated by a physiotherapist with specialist training?

All physiotherapists have spent at least three years getting their degree and becoming chartered physiotherapists. They then start a period of training where they move between posts offering different experience. Once they decide what area they wish to specialise in, they take a job in that field and often start attending post-graduate courses to gain further expertise. In physiotherapy, the major speciality that is likely to be involved in treating you after a stroke is neurology – neuro-physiotherapy. There are only a few therapists who spend their whole time treating people who have had a stroke, although as the number of stroke units increases so the number of stroke specialist therapists will also increase. It is important that your therapy is co-ordinated by someone with expertise in neuro-physiotherapy and that that person is part of a multi-disciplinary team who meet regularly to plan and monitor your rehabilitation. The day-to-day therapy may well be given by a more junior therapist and that is perfectly acceptable, provided they are being supervised.

Do some types of physiotherapy treatment work better than others?

Not that we know about at the moment. There are two major schools of thought in the therapy world. One is based on principles defined by a husband and wife team called Bobath, and the other one is named after two Australian therapists called Carr and Shepherd. In fact, there isn't all that much difference between the two schools of therapy, although each has very strong advocates, arguing that theirs is the only correct way of doing business. Many physiotherapists adopt a pragmatic approach and use what they consider to be the best bits of each technique appropriate for an individual person with stroke. The important thing about physiotherapy is that it is provided by optimistic enthusiasts who enjoy their job and whose primary objective in life is to get you better.

The physiotherapist keeps telling me to slow down and to do only the exercises she has shown me. I feel she is holding back my recovery. What can I do?

It is very important that you regain as much normal function as possible, so take the physiotherapist's advice. Although you might be able to get there faster, this could be at the cost of quality of movement. For example, you might be able to get walking soon – but with a limp. If you take your time, you will probably walk without a limp. This is not just a cosmetic difference. Walking badly for a few years can end up with your getting back pain or even arthritis in your hips and knees. Obviously you want to make as much progress as possible as quickly as possible but it really is a mistake to try to run before you can walk. Make sure the physiotherapist explains to you what she is doing and why. Get her to tell you what she expects you to be able to learn this week. Don't try to get her to read too far into the future, because that is a bit like long-term weather forecasting: more often wrong than right.

If you really aren't happy with your physiotherapist, it should be possible to get a second opinion – either from another therapist in the hospital or by your paying for a private physiotherapist to come in and do an assessment.

I've had strapping put round my shoulder. What is this supposed to do?

The shoulder is particularly vulnerable to injury early after a stroke. It is a joint that depends heavily on the normal working of the muscles to keep the ends of the two bones together. If the muscles stop working, the humerus (the bone of the upper arm) and the scapula (the shoulder blade) can move apart. This is called *subluxation* or *partial dislocation*. If the joint stretches in this way, the capsule round the joint and the ligaments can become inflamed and painful. In most cases a painful shoulder after a stroke can be prevented by:

- treating the arm with care,

- positioning it carefully,

- never allowing the arm to hang down.

Some therapists strap the shoulder with bandages. Although it has not been proven to work, it seems likely that it will have two effects: first, it will help keep the joint in the correct position; and secondly – probably more important – it will act as a reminder to you, your relatives and the staff that the shoulder needs careful handling. The Bobath Cuff is one of the various straps and slings that have been devised. They all aim to work in similar ways but with no evidence that any one is better than another.

A 'frozen shoulder' is one that is painful or difficult to move because of damage to the ligaments and capsule round the joint. It can take many months to settle down and can seriously set back attempts to regain normal function in the arm. This is an instance where prevention is clearly better than cure.

**I don't seem to be achieving much now with the physio-
therapy. How long is it worth persevering with it?**

It is worth carrying on with physiotherapy as long as you are
continuing to make progress. The most rapid recovery is usually
in the first few weeks after the stroke. After that, change is slower
but can continue for a long time. The pattern of recovery differs
from person to person: your recovery will depend on the size, type
and position of the stroke, what you were like physically and
mentally before the stroke, and how you are coping emotionally
after the stroke. It is difficult to generalise but below are some
basic principles for you.

- Don't give up too soon. Even if there is not much sign of
  improving muscle function, if you are improving in other
  ways there is still the potential for improvement with
  physiotherapy.

- If you and the physiotherapist decide between you that the
  time has come to stop therapy, there should always be an
  easy way for you to be reviewed if things start to change,
  whether for better or worse.

- Don't keep on with physiotherapy indefinitely. There comes
  a point when nothing more can be gained. In fact, at that
  point it can become counter-productive to keep going. All
  that is being done is to keep showing you what you can't
  do, and this can be dispiriting. Keeping on with the
  physiotherapy might prevent you from coming to terms
  with problems that are not going to go away. If you
  genuinely reach a plateau in rehabilitation, it is important
  to recognise that fact and start to find ways round the
  problems that you are left with.

Muscle stiffness or weakness

Even though I have got some movement back, I can't use my arm because it feels so stiff. The physio says this is due to 'spasticity'. What is it and what treatment can I have for it?

Spasticity is the medical term for muscles that are abnormally stiff. Initially after a stroke your muscles will be floppy (flaccid) as well as weak. For example, if your arm or leg is lifted and put through a range of movements, there will seem to be very little resistance. Within a few days after the stroke, even if no strength has returned, the muscles usually start to stiffen. When someone tries to move the arm or leg for you, it will be much more difficult. Several factors can make the stiffness worse:

- If your body is kept in the wrong positions for a long time either in bed or when you are sitting in a chair.

- If you try to do everything with your unaffected side, this can cause the stiffness to increase on the paralysed side.

- If you are uncomfortable or in pain.

- If you develop any other medical problems, such as an infection.

It is very important that the stiffness of your muscles is not allowed to become too severe, because if the muscles are very stiff it will become very difficult for you to move them once your strength starts returning. The treatment lies in recognising that there is a problem and then doing everything possible to prevent it. Within a few minutes of starting a treatment session, a skilled physiotherapist can reduce stiffness in muscles by getting your posture right and manipulating your limbs. It is important that the physiotherapist tells the nurses about how you should be moved and positioned correctly.

If the stiffness is not treated early, the joints and muscles can get so stiff that it becomes impossible for anyone to move the joint – a *contracture*. Once this has happened, it is quite difficult to get the joint functioning again.

The physiotherapist has asked the doctor to prescribe a drug to try to reduce the stiffness in my muscles. Do they really help?

Sometimes it is helpful to treat you with drugs to try to reduce the stiffness, although they don't always work. The three main drugs used are baclofen, dantrolene and tizanidine. You will usually start at a low dose and gradually build up, so you may not notice much benefit at first. The physiotherapist and the doctor will be carefully monitoring the effects of the drug to make sure that it is working and not causing any unacceptable side effects. The main side effects of all three drugs are drowsiness and, sometimes, confusion.

Another problem that can occasionally arise is that the drugs can be too effective. If you can walk despite having very weak muscles, you will depend on the muscles in your leg being stiff enough to help hold you up. If all the stiffness is taken away, you may find that you don't have enough strength to stay upright. These drugs therefore need to be used only under the careful supervision of your stroke team.

The muscles in my hand are very tight, so that I can't straighten them out. I've been told that injections with botulinum toxin are helpful. How can I get them?

Botulinum toxin is a powerful poison that blocks the action of the nerves on the muscle. Taken in large quantities it rapidly causes death. Injecting very small amounts into the muscles can reduce their stiffness, and can be helpful in the sort of situation you describe. There is little point having it unless there is significant strength in your hand muscles that will be released by reducing the stiffness. If the conditions are right, it is worth trying.

Not all centres in the UK are experienced at using botulinum toxin. It is given by several injections at sites that are usually determined by the use of *electromyography*. This is a technique where a needle in the muscle records the electrical activity and can identify where the nerve is connected to the muscle. The effect of the botulinum toxin lasts only about three months and the drug is incredibly expensive, which is probably why the treatment is not widely available. Your consultant and the physiotherapist will be able to advise you whether it would be appropriate for you and where you might be able to get it. It is very important that the injections are combined with physiotherapy to maximise any benefits you will get.

Is botulinum toxin any use for the stiffness in my legs?

Unfortunately, botulinum toxin is really only of any use for small muscles. Large muscles such as those in the leg would require too much of the drug and too many injections for it to be feasible, either medically or financially.

Several of my joints have become so stiff that I can't move them, which makes it difficult for me to even sit comfortably. What can be done to straighten out my arms and legs?

The treatment of these *contractures* is extremely difficult. Really the only way to tackle them is to put splints on your arms and legs to stretch them out. The physiotherapist or occupational therapist will make splints that you wear for as much of the day and night as you can tolerate. As each joint starts to stretch out, a new splint will be made that stretches it even further. The splinting is combined with physiotherapy. It can be very painful to try to stretch a fixed joint and you will probably need quite strong pain-killers before your treatment session. The process is slow and there is no guarantee of success. If it doesn't work and you can't even sit comfortably, it is sometimes feasible to have an operation to cut the tendons, which are the fibrous bands that connect the muscle to the bone, and stretch the joint out under anaesthetic. This treatment is used only as a last resort.

I had my stroke three months ago and I still feel generally weak and tired. Would it be safe for me to start going back to my local fitness centre?

You should ask your doctor and physiotherapist first, to make sure that it won't harm your recovery. Generally, it is probably an excellent idea to start thinking about regaining general physical fitness. It can make you feel much healthier and be an important stage in getting you back to a normal life. The fitness instructor at the centre might need a letter from your doctor before they take you on. Once they have this authorisation, they can often devise excellent programmes suited to your situation.

If you don't feel like using the fancy machines in the gym, think about trying swimming, which can be an excellent way of regaining fitness, even if you have some weakness of one side of your body.

What is functional electrical stimulation?

One of the problems after a stroke is that the muscles get weak because they are not being used. Even without a stroke, just lying in bed or sitting in a chair not moving around much will cause your muscles to get weak. To try to prevent this from happening and to stimulate the recovery of muscle function, a technique called functional electrical stimulation (FES) has been tried. This involves using electrodes placed on the skin overlying a muscle or nerve to stimulate contraction of the muscle. Although this can prevent your muscle from wasting, unfortunately it does not really seem to help in terms of improving the use of your arm or leg. FES is being tested in some research studies, so perhaps more information will become available over the next few years.

I have lost a lot of strength as a result of doing very little since my stroke. I am keen to build up my muscles again. Could I take some of the drugs that athletes use?

The drugs that some athletes use (illegally for sport) are the anabolic steroids (the male hormones) and human growth hormone. These steroids could be very harmful by causing damage to the heart, and there is little to suggest that they would be useful in your situation. There is research going on to see what medical role (or roles) there is for growth hormone. It is not licensed to be used to rebuild strength after illness and the early research findings do not really encourage the belief that it is likely to be of much use. Much safer and probably more effective is a properly planned exercise programme.

Aids and equipment

I think that I'd get going quicker if the therapist gave me a walking frame. Why won't she?

Don't be in too much of a rush. For some people, a walking frame is the correct solution and enables them to get back to walking when they otherwise wouldn't. But surely it would be better to be able to walk without a frame, even if it takes you a little longer? Your rehabilitation is a balance between what is possible and what is ideal. If your therapist is not keen to give you a frame now, it is very likely that she thinks you won't need one in the long term. If you use a frame at this stage, you could get into bad habits and even become psychologically dependent on the frame to the point where you feel too frightened to walk without it. Take the advice of your therapist. She really is in the best position to advise you.

We're working hard to get me moving about but it's quite difficult. Will I have to use a walking stick when I go home?

It is often quite late in rehabilitation before it is possible to know exactly what the best walking aid will be for an individual. The aim is always to get people to function with as little in the way of aids as possible, and then to use the simplest aid there is. So the therapist will always choose the walking stick in preference to a frame if at all possible. You may find that you need a stick in some situations and can manage without it in others. Typically, you'll be able to manage well indoors without any help, but find you need a stick when walking outside because of uneven ground and the lack of things to hold onto if you begin to feel unsteady. If you need a walking stick, it must be adjusted to you. Never use one left to you by your grandfather, or one belonging to a neighbour, without first checking it with your therapist. It must be the correct length, and must always have a good-quality rubber tip (ferrule) to prevent the stick from sliding away from you on slippery surfaces. (Check the ferrule regularly, as they get worn down, resulting in the stick no longer having a good grip on the floor. Your physiotherapist should be able to give you a new one.)

The type of stick you are given will depend on why you are using it. Some people need the stick to help support some of their weight when walking; others are given a stick to help them balance rather than to take weight. In my view [AR] all walking aids should be available only on prescription in the same way as medicines. An incorrect walking stick can be as dangerous as a wrong drug or one taken incorrectly.

There doesn't seem to be much equipment in the gym. Would I not do better if I were somewhere a bit more high tech?

The three most important pieces of equipment in the gym are the physiotherapist's brain and hands. If you visited physiotherapy departments elsewhere in Europe, you would probably be struck by how much more equipment there was compared with the UK, but there is very little evidence to suggest that they provide any benefit. Sometimes, if there is a shortage of trained therapists, the equipment can provide a substitute, but certainly don't judge your physiotherapy department by how many gadgets it has.

I'd like to try hydrotherapy. Is it helpful after stroke?

Hydrotherapy is the term for physiotherapy in a pool filled with warm water. Being in water provides you with support: your body doesn't feel so heavy and if you have weak limbs they may be easier to move. It can also be easier to keep your balance. Not all hospitals will have a hydrotherapy pool; there are differences of opinion about what their role is, they are expensive to build and maintain, and there have to be enough therapists in the department to be able to offer the treatment. If your hospital does have a pool, there are certain situations where it can be helpful after stroke. If your arm or leg is weak and stiff, it could be easier to get it moving in the warm water. It might also be useful in getting you to stand upright as part of your balance training.

You will not normally be able to use the pool if you have any incontinence, an open wound or an infection – for obvious reasons.

Often I feel too tired to go to the gym and I send the porter away. Am I doing myself long-term harm?

It really is important to start with your rehabilitation as early as possible after the stroke. The early days are times when the limbs can become very stiff if they are not moved and positioned correctly. Lying in bed all the time will not help you get back your sense of balance. It will be more difficult for you to eat properly if you are in bed at mealtimes, and staying in bed for too long can be dangerous – there is a greater chance of blood clots forming in your legs and of your developing a chest infection. For all these reasons it is important to force yourself to get out of bed to go down to the gym. Overwhelming tiredness in the early stages is very common, and you are not alone in wanting to spend your time in bed, sleeping. Get the physiotherapists and nurses to co-ordinate their work so that you are not got out of bed, washed and dressed until just before your appointment in the gym. Agree with the nurses when you will be sitting out during the day and when you can go back to bed for a sleep.

A friend brought me a ball to squeeze to help build up the strength in my arm but the physiotherapist told me it would do more harm than good. Is he right?

In most instances after a stroke, it is not a good idea to try to improve strength in the hand by squeezing a ball. Weakness is not the only problem that needs to be overcome. The muscles also become stiff (spastic) and ball squeezing can make the stiffness worse. There will be things that you and your friend can do to help you in your recovery. Get your friend to talk to the physiotherapist or attend one of your therapy sessions to find out useful exercises that you can be doing in between treatment sessions.

Wheelchairs

If I need a wheelchair will I have to buy it, and who will organise it for me?

Wheelchairs are provided free by the NHS to anyone who needs one. There will be a district wheelchair service, responsible for assessing people and then prescribing the appropriate chair and cushion. If it is decided that you should have a wheelchair, it is very important that it meets your needs.

- Do you need a chair that will be pushed around by someone else or one that you are going to propel yourself?

- If you are going to have a chair that you can move on your own, does it need to be adapted to use with just one arm?

- Is it mainly for outdoor use or just around the house?

- Do you have special needs that might mean that you should have a very lightweight chair?

- Would you benefit from an electrically operated chair?

Having decided on the type of chair, it must be made to fit you

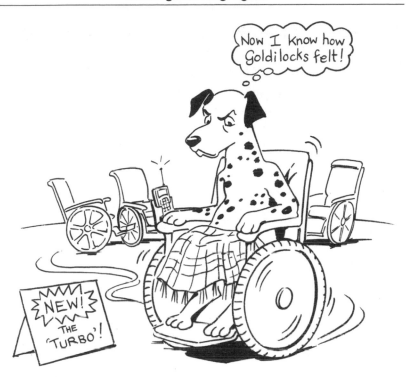

exactly. Too big and it won't give you the necessary support and may not fit through your doors at home. Too small and you'll end up with sores over your hips. If you are going to be sitting in the chair all day, you will need a special pressure-relieving cushion to prevent pressure sores.

The wheelchair service, unfortunately, does not have unlimited resources and often the type of chair provided will be one of the very basic models. Money may well be able to buy more. It is possible that the wheelchair service can give you a voucher towards the cost of buying a wheelchair privately. If you do wish to invest in a chair, the wheelchair service or your occupational therapist may be able to give you advice. Alternatively, most areas have a Disabled Living Centre not too far away where the chairs will be available to try out.

If you just need a wheelchair for a short time, the Red Cross sometimes has them available for hire.

I'd like an electric wheelchair. Will I be entitled to one?

Electric wheelchairs or scooters for use outside are not usually provided by the NHS wheelchair service, so you would probably have to obtain one privately. They can cost several thousand pounds, although there is a second-hand market where they can be bought for considerably less. You will also need to consider where you would keep it: it must be somewhere dry, secure and accessible. The occupational therapist can tell you whether you'll be able to use an electric wheelchair. Just as with driving a car, you need to be competent to drive one, as they can be quite dangerous if driven into someone.

The major reason why people get turned down for an electric chair is that they have lost their sight on one side. The chairs are, however, quite simple to use and with a bit of practice even the most unlikely seeming people have mastered the controls. Electric wheelchairs can be tremendously liberating. Having perhaps struggled for months trying to walk a few steps, now you can get down to the shop to buy your own newspaper or into the kitchen to make a sandwich.

I don't want to have to rely on others to take me about. What about those electric cars for going down to the shops?

Most of the electric wheelchairs provided by the wheelchair service are solely for use indoors. If you want to use an electric chair to go to the shops, to visit friends or nip down to the pub, you will have to invest in an outdoor version. These are not usually provided free. They are expensive, costing upwards of £2,000. There is a second-hand market and you may be able to pick one up more cheaply. Again, don't consider buying one until you have consulted an expert, such as the occupational therapist, about whether you will be able to use it and what sort to get. You can get advice on how to use one from a mobility centre. You will also need to think about where you will keep it. If you are going to use it to go to the pub, don't forget that, although you don't need a licence to drive an electric car, drink–drive laws still apply!

Complementary therapies

Does acupuncture help? How can I organise it?

There is contradictory evidence as to whether acupuncture does help after a stroke. Some research trials have suggested that it does speed recovery a little. However, in recent trials, the people who had the acupuncture did no better than those who didn't have it. In none of the people studied did it cause any harm, though. If you are keen to try it, our advice would be to give it a go. It is important to use an acupuncturist who is properly qualified. Contact the British Acupuncture Council (address in Appendix 1) for details of practitioners in your area. It is occasionally available on the NHS.

What about aromatherapy or massage?

There is even less hard scientific evidence to support the use of massage, aromatherapy, shiatsu or the other sorts of complementary treatments than there is for acupuncture. It is quite likely that your doctors will be rather sceptical about such treatments, but don't allow them to put you off unless they can give some good reasons. There is a lot of conventional medicine that is not strongly supported by much evidence either! A lack of evidence either means it doesn't work or that no one has yet conducted a trial to test it, and very few of the massage-type treatments have so far been tested.

It is unlikely they will do any harm but it would be important to discuss with your physiotherapist whether there are certain types that might interfere with what he or she is doing. If you do decide to try out some of the complementary therapies, it would be wise to clarify at the beginning exactly what they are attempting to achieve. Then carefully monitor whether the treatment is achieving its goals or not. It is possible to spend very large amounts of money with little to show for it at the end.

4
Swallowing and nutrition

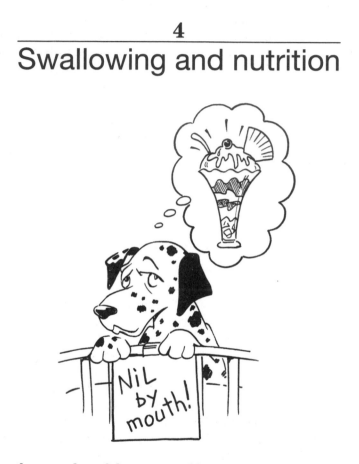

Just as the muscles of the arms and legs can be weak and difficult to control after a stroke, so can the muscles controlling speech and swallowing. The swallowing mechanism is incredibly delicate, involving hundreds of muscles. Disturbance of any of these muscles can affect the safety of swallowing. It used to be believed that only strokes affecting the brainstem or both sides of the brain would damage swallowing but it is now known that *any* stroke can result in an unsafe swallow.

The mouth and throat are the normal routes to the stomach and the lungs. When we eat and drink, it is essential that none of the food or drink goes down our windpipe to enter our lungs – called *aspiration*. If this happens, food may block the airway or get into the lung, allowing infection to enter, possibly causing pneumonia. Aspiration can occur without the person coughing, spluttering or showing any other outward signs of a problem and because of this it is essential to check swallowing safety. By making sure that everyone who has a stroke is properly checked to see whether their swallowing is safe, many people have been identified who, without proper attention, would have been at risk of developing pneumonia.

Swallowing

My husband has a 'nil by mouth' sign at the end of his bed. Why?

It is likely that your husband has been identified as being at risk of aspirating, as explained above, and has quite correctly been kept 'nil by mouth'. It is important that the nurses let you know about this so that you and any other visitors do not tempt your husband with irresistible tasty morsels.

While he is 'nil by mouth', it is important to maintain good oral hygiene, so that his mouth doesn't become dry, sore and infected. Brushing his teeth regularly, cleaning his dentures (if any), keeping his mouth moist with wet swabs provided by the nursing staff and putting petroleum jelly (e.g. Vaseline) around his lips and giving him ice cubes to suck will all be helpful. There is little worse than a mouth caked with dried saliva and mucus from the chest and nose: it tastes awful and your breath starts to smell. It also affects your appetite and can generally make you feel wretched. Mouth care needs to be done several times a day – it might be something the nurses would appreciate the family giving some help with when they visit.

The doctor has told me that my son mustn't eat or drink anything because it might go down the wrong way and cause pneumonia. How long can he go without food, and when will he be able to swallow again?

Most of us have at least a couple of weeks' food reserves stored in our body and can go with little nutrition for that length of time without doing ourselves much harm. We cannot, however, go for more than a couple of days without water. Most people who have swallowing difficulties after a stroke recover their swallowing mechanism within the first few days. By two weeks over two-thirds of them are swallowing safely. So the doctors usually decide to give fluids by drip (through a tube into a vein) and not worry too much about the lack of food; the hope is that the swallowing reflex will recover and make it unnecessary to feed by tube.

Your son's swallowing mechanism should be checked regularly, and advice given by a speech and language therapist as to what progress is being made. When recovery starts, it will probably be safer for him to swallow thickened drinks rather than normal drinks. Special thickeners are available that can easily be added to any liquid for this purpose. While thickened tea or Guinness may not be everyone's idea of an appetising drink, it is likely that within a few days he will be back on the real thing. At first, his food may need to be pureed. As his swallowing gets better, he may move on to soft foods such as fish or mashed potato before returning to a normal diet.

The doctor is talking about possibly using a nasogastric tube or a gastrostomy for my wife. Are they necessary and, if so, which one is better?

A *nasogastric tube* is a tube that goes up the nose, into the back of the throat and down into the stomach. Although it can be a bit uncomfortable while the tube is being inserted, once in place people soon forget it is there. Unlike the larger nasogastric tubes used to empty the stomach, the feeding tubes are not much wider than a piece of spaghetti.

A *gastrostomy tube* (sometimes known as a PEG tube – for 'percutaneous endoscopic gastrostomy') is a fine tube that is inserted through the abdomen directly into the stomach for the purposes of feeding. The usual way of placing the gastrostomy tube is to pass an endoscope down the throat into the stomach (a gastroscopy), which allows the doctor to shine a bright light from the inside of the stomach. This light is used to guide where to insert a small needle directly into the stomach. (Local anaesthetic is used to numb the skin before the needle is inserted.) The gastrostomy tube is passed over the needle into the stomach and held in place with a balloon inflated at the end of the tube. The whole procedure takes only a few minutes and should not be too uncomfortable. Sometimes ultrasound is used instead of the endoscope to identify where to insert the tube.

If your wife has a problem with swallowing safely, tube feeding should be considered. As mentioned in the answer above, one of the options is just to use a drip for a few days in the hope that her ability to swallow will recover. If it doesn't or if it is important to provide nutrition early, the doctor will decide which sort of tube to opt for – both have advantages and disadvantages.

The nasogastric tube

- This is easy to insert but also falls out very easily – there are times when the tube comes out so often that it is never in long enough to get any food down!

- Some people hate having the tube inserted, while others find that it irritates when it is in place.

- Having a tube going down the throat could possibly increase the risk of infection getting into the lungs.

The gastrostomy tube

- The big advantage is that it very rarely falls out.

- Once in, it is less irritating – even with people who are very restless.

- Because it is hidden under clothes, it tends not to be fiddled with.

- The major disadvantage is that it requires a small cut to be made in the abdomen, which can become infected.

- It also requires a further gastroscopy to remove it. This involves passing a tube into the stomach which enables the doctor to detach the tube from the stomach wall.

What happens if you put in a feeding tube and my husband never improves? He'd hate being kept alive like this if he is not going to get better.

Sometimes there is a worry that artificial feeding will be the only thing keeping the person alive when there is absolutely no prospect of their recovering any useful function, and that there will be an ethical dilemma if it is felt that the tube should be removed. In fact, guidance from the British Medical Association says that ethically there is no difference between the decision not to insert a tube in the first place and the decision to withdraw one that is already in place.

There has recently been a report on the results of a very large trial that attempted to answer the questions:

- how soon should tube feeding start after a stroke?

- what sort of tube should be used: a nasogastric tube or a gastrostomy tube?

Even though many thousands of patients were included in the study, the results didn't give any clear-cut answers, as there weren't any big differences in the outcomes between any of the groups in the trial. My [AR] practice is now to start feeding through a nasogastric tube as soon as possible, if the person can't swallow safely, unless the stroke is so severe that recovery is remote. If a tube is likely to be needed for several weeks, or if the nasogastric tube isn't tolerated, I recommend a gastrostomy tube.

Is there any therapy available that will speed up getting my swallowing back to normal?

Unfortunately, there is no treatment to speed up the recovery of swallowing, although some therapists claim that it helps to stimulate the throat with ice.

How quickly your swallowing recovers will depend on the size and position of your stroke, and on the extent to which the control of swallowing is represented on both sides of your brain. In some people the nerve cells controlling their swallowing reflex are almost exclusively in one half of the brain, while in others control is divided between the right and left sides. For people with control on one side, a stroke affecting that side of the brain will severely damage their ability to swallow. For those with control on both sides, a stroke affecting just the right or the left hemisphere will not cause significant problems.

A small study has suggested that, even in people at risk of liquids going into their lungs, it does not do any harm to allow them pure water. This finding is still controversial, but is not altogether surprising. A little water, even if aspirated into the lungs, may not do much harm. And even people who are given nothing by mouth are probably still getting saliva in their lungs. At least if water is allowed, there is less likely to be infection in their mouth that might spread to their lungs.

My brother just isn't eating enough and has lost an awful lot of weight. Do you have any suggestions?

Even without difficulties in swallowing, losing weight after a stroke is common. As with any illness, your brother may have lost his appetite. If he was drowsy when he was first in hospital, he will have eaten less. Hospital food is not always appetising and if there are difficulties with the mechanics of eating, such as problems holding cutlery, this will also contribute to his lower calorie intake.

The solution to weight loss is to find out which of these factors was responsible. Loss of appetite is the most difficult factor to resolve. Oddly enough, when someone has not been eating for a time, their appetite can disappear altogether and only reappear when they start forcing themselves to eat. Encouragement and offering your brother food that he used to like most might work. Giving him energy-rich foods, such as cream or full-fat ice cream on top of the desserts, can increase calorie intake enormously without his needing to consume large volumes of food. Don't be frightened to bring in food from home if you think that he is more likely to eat this than hospital food. Check first with the staff that there are no special dietary requirements such as a need for puree or soft consistency.

The doctors or dietitians can prescribe energy- and protein-rich drinks, which are sometimes more acceptable than normal diets. The dietitian will be able to provide skilled advice on your brother's food requirements and how these might best be provided. Vitamin and mineral supplements in tablet form may be required if his loss of appetite goes on for long. An option that might be considered would be to feed your brother through a tube, either nasogastric or gastrostomy, until his normal appetite returns. Tube feeding at night and then encouraging normal eating during the day is a solution that has been used successfully.

If your brother's problem is that eating is too difficult because of a physical disability, the occupational therapist may be able to help. Giving him cutlery that he can use with one hand, using a 'plate guard' that stops the food being pushed off the plate and making sure that he is sitting up rather than lying in bed at mealtimes are all important. If he needs assistance with eating, it will be very useful if you can arrange visits so that friends and relatives are available to help at appropriate times.

I won't be able to cope with my husband at home if he can't eat or drink and has to have a tube feed. What will happen to him?

There are many people who live at home despite depending on tube feeding, and this even applies to people who live alone. In fact, managing a tube feed is very easy, and the community nurse can provide any help and support required. All that is needed is to connect the tube from a bottle of feed to the end of the gastrostomy or nasogastric tube and open the tap to allow the liquid to run in. There is very little that can go wrong. It is not like feeding directly into the blood stream, where getting air or infection into the system can be dangerous. You don't have to watch the liquid running in and it doesn't matter if the bottle of food runs out.

In some ways it is actually much simpler than preparing special food or helping someone who has difficulty swallowing. The problems that can be encountered are infection around the tube site and the tube getting blocked. Neither of these is an emergency, but you should ask your GP or nurse to call. If, despite everything, you feel you won't be able to cope, the only alternative is to consider with your husband whether he should go into a nursing home. This is obviously a big step to take. Think about giving home a try first; if it does prove too difficult, a nursing home is always an option later.

Nutrition and diet

I'm overweight and for years have been trying to lose weight and yet they are still bullying me to eat. What is wrong with them?

After a stroke it is important to maintain an adequate intake of protein and energy, to help regain the strength that you may have lost. Although in the longer run it will be sensible to lose weight, this is not the time to do it. A healthy diet containing the right balance of vitamins, minerals, protein, carbohydrates and fat is necessary during any illness, and stroke is no exception. The problem with dieting now is that you will lose weight by losing some of your muscle as well as your fat stores. You need every ounce of muscle at the moment to take part in your rehabilitation; in fact, you need to be building up your muscle to regain your independence.

Once you are over the initial 'acute' phase of the stroke, it will be worth seeing the dietitian. At that stage you should aim to get

onto a diet that will gradually bring your weight down to a
reasonable level. Being overweight will make it more difficult for
your legs to carry you and will put an additional strain on your
heart and lungs.

I've put on a lot of weight since the stroke even though I hardly eat anything. What is it due to?

This is a frequent complaint and is usually due to your becoming
less active yet continuing to eat the same amount (or more). The
best solution is to find some sort of exercise you can do that will
both make you feel physically fitter and increase the amount of
food you are burning up. This doesn't need to be anything very
vigorous. If you can't get up and exercise by walking, you can
burn up quite a lot of energy by repeatedly lifting your arm and
leg up and down. Doing it to music usually makes it seem less of
a chore. If you combine this with a diet that reduces your calorie
intake by a little every day, you will begin to feel fitter and start
losing weight.

It is worth seeing a dietitian who will be able to go through
your diet with you in detail and suggest ways that you will be able
to eat more healthily.

Does cholesterol play a part in causing stroke?

The link between cholesterol and stroke is not as strong as that
between cholesterol and heart attack. If cholesterol and the low-
density lipoproteins (LDLs) are present in your blood in large
quantities, they result in the build-up of fatty deposits in the walls
of the arteries – which makes them more likely to be blocked off
with blood clot.

There is no logical reason why there should be much
difference between stroke and heart disease, and some of the
large trials designed mainly to study the effect of lowering
cholesterol on heart disease have also shown a reduction in the
incidence of stroke. Increasingly, therefore, doctors who
specialise in treating people who have had stroke try hard to
bring cholesterol levels down as low as possible. This is usually

achieved by a combination of diet and one of the 'statin' drugs such as pravastatin or simvastatin. There are lots of similar drugs that act in much the same way and they are probably as good as each other. It is certainly worth having your cholesterol measured and then discussing with your doctor whether any treatment is desirable.

I've been told to cut down on the amount of fat in my diet. Can you recommend the best way to do this?

What you should or should not eat varies between individuals. For everyone, not just people who have had a stroke, it is sensible to try to reduce the amount of cholesterol in their diet. This means reducing both the amount of animal fat and the amount of total fat in your diet.

- If you are cooking, use vegetable oils such as corn oil or olive oil rather than butter or lard.

- Avoid frying food. Whenever possible, boil or steam your food. Grilling is better than frying, and it often tastes better.

- If you can bear it, switch from butter to soft margarine on your bread.

- Limit the number of eggs you eat each week to two or three. The yolks especially are very rich in cholesterol.

- Reduce the amount of fatty meat you eat and instead eat fish or lean meat such as poultry. If you are eating pork, beef or lamb, cut off all the fat before you start cooking it.

- Avoid processed meat such as sausages, salami, burgers of all sorts and meat pies.

- Shellfish are quite rich in cholesterol, but better than many meats. Eat them in moderation.

- Drink semi-skimmed or skimmed milk rather than full-cream milk, and avoid cream. If you do like cream, try switching to yoghurt or fromage frais.

- Avoid eating full-fat cheeses, such as Cheddar and cream cheese, and try lower fat cheeses such as cottage cheese, some of the soft cheeses such as Brie and Camembert. Try to reduce the total amount of cheese you eat.

- Eat more fish, which is low in saturated fat. Try to have fish on your diet at least twice a week. Experiment with different sorts of fish. Sometimes the ugliest ones are the ones that taste best!

- Instead of ice cream, try frozen yoghurt or sorbets.

- Avoid lashings of peanut butter.

Diets are made to be broken, especially if there is a special occasion. No one can be good all the time, so don't feel too guilty when you sin; rather, enjoy it and get back onto the straight and narrow tomorrow. Then look forward to the next special occasion . . . but not too soon!

The doctor has told me that my cholesterol level is too high. What should it be?

The evidence seems to suggest that the lower the cholesterol the better. You should be aiming for a total cholesterol of less than 5 millimoles per litre of blood (5mmol/l), although the risks of heart disease, and stroke, continue to fall as the cholesterol level falls. The 'bad' cholesterol is the LDL (low-density lipoprotein); if your total cholesterol is high, your doctor will want to check the level of the LDL. You should be aiming to get your LDL cholesterol level down to below 3.2mmol/l.

We're trying to get my cholesterol down. How often should I have it measured?

Your cholesterol will usually be measured when you are first assessed after your stroke. If the level is high, you will be given dietary advice and probably some medication. There is little point measuring it again until you have been on the diet for about three months.

Is my high cholesterol due solely to what I eat?

Some people inherit their tendency to high cholesterol from their parents. In these cases the level is usually very high (above 8mmol/l) and there is often a strong family history of heart disease and stroke. If this is the case with you, you should be started straight away on a cholesterol-lowering drug and be referred to your local lipid clinic where the treatment can be carefully monitored.

Do the drugs that are used to treat high cholesterol have any side effects?

The drugs that are most often used to lower cholesterol are the statins. These drugs seldom have side effects but in a small proportion of people can cause muscle pains, a rash, indigestion and, occasionally, reduced sex drive. If you get any of these side effects, stop taking the drug and go back to see your doctor. He or she will be able to prescribe an alternative.

I'm 76 years old and have had a mild stroke. Is there really any point at my age worrying about my diet?

Your natural life expectancy at 76 is about another 10 years. It really is worth making sure that the remaining years of your life are spent fit and active rather than in a disabled state as a result of another stroke. We don't think it makes any difference what your age is. You should be doing everything you can to stop yourself having another stroke, and if that means changing your diet or taking a tablet to lower your cholesterol, so be it.

My sister is always going on about too much salt. Should I reduce the amount of salt I eat?

Yes. A lot of salt in the diet is linked to high blood pressure, and even if your blood pressure is normal it won't do any harm to get it a bit lower. Eating lots of salt gets to be a bit of a habit. People who succeed in cutting it down usually report that after a few weeks they no longer find they want any more. If possible, gradually stop putting salt in your cooking and try to switch from using processed food, which often contains very large amounts of salt. At the very least, stop adding salt to your food once it is on the plate. If you really can't manage without salt and other sorts of seasoning aren't good enough, you can buy salt substitute that is made of potassium chloride rather than sodium chloride (available from supermarkets or chemist/pharmacist shops). Make sure that your doctor knows you are using it.

How can I lose weight? I really don't eat much.

Life isn't fair. Some people can eat vast amounts without getting fat while others seem to get fat just by thinking about food. If you are one of the latter group, comfort yourself with the thought that your body is clearly much more efficient than the others and that if you get stuck on a desert island with no food you will survive much longer than the thin people!

Fat is the tissue that the body uses to store energy for times when food might be scarce. What you eat is either used to provide energy immediately or put into store for later, or it is passed straight out in the faeces. If you eat only as much as your body needs, there is no way in which you can gain weight. If you eat less than you need, your body has to start using up its fat reserves and you will lose weight. So there are two ways of losing weight: either eat less or increase your energy requirements by exercising more . . . but without compensating by eating a few extra chocolate bars! The best solution is to do a combination of both.

Dieting is not easy. There is no magic solution – if there were, there would not have been so many hundreds of books written on the subject, each with their own miraculous diet. The key is to do it slowly, by small adjustments to your diet that you will be able to maintain over a long period. Start by keeping a food diary for a week, listing everything you eat or drink. You have to be honest with yourself: one reason why people don't succeed at dieting is that they fool themselves, almost as if eating something with their eyes closed doesn't count! Sit down with your food diary at the end of the week and decide what you could do without. Maybe switching to low-fat milk, or not having that biscuit mid-morning. Perhaps one less pint of beer or limit the chocolate bingeing to once a week. Artificial sweeteners instead of sugar, sugar-free chewing gum instead of sweets. Keep it to a fairly small change that is not too painful. Then weigh yourself once a week. If you can lose one kilogram a month, by the end of the first year you will have lost 12 kilograms or nearly two stone. The problem with diets that are designed to make you lose a stone in a month is that they are impossible to maintain, and you almost always put the weight back on within a short time.

Exercising may be more difficult, particularly if your mobility has been impaired as a result of the stroke. If you are less active than you used to be, you will first have to reduce your energy intake to prevent yourself from gaining weight. The sort of exercise that you are able to do will depend on how your stroke has affected you. Consider joining a local fitness club where there will be experts able to advise on what sort of exercises will be appropriate for you. There may be particular sorts of equipment that are suited to your needs. Health clubs often require a letter from your doctor, giving some information about you and saying what exercise is appropriate for you. Even if you have been confined to a chair, it is still possible to stay physically fit using your unaffected arm and leg.

Swimming is a very good way of getting fit, especially if you have some weakness on one side. It may take some courage at

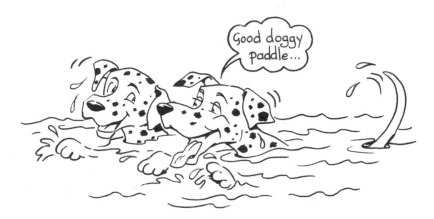

first to get into the water, but if you could swim before your stroke it is very likely you will still be able to, even if you don't look quite so elegant. For the first time, go to a pool that has a very shallow end or a children's pool just to get used to how to float again, and go with someone who can help you if necessary. Swimming in the sea can be even easier because of the added buoyancy provided by the salt water. So don't dismiss the idea of a holiday at the beach. It could be good for you.

All my family is big-boned. Now I'm told that I'm overweight. How can they tell?

The way that doctors and dietitians check this is to use the Body Mass Index (BMI). Weight on its own doesn't mean much without knowing how tall you are. The BMI is calculated using the formula

$$\text{BMI} = \frac{\text{weight in kilograms}}{(\text{height in metres})^2}$$

For example, if you weigh 70 kg and are 1.7 metres tall, your BMI will be:

$$\frac{70}{(1.7)^2} = \frac{70}{2.9} = 24.1$$

Your doctor will be able to calculate your BMI for you, if you don't have a calculator; or you can work it out from the chart in Figure 6. The normal BMI is 20–25. A BMI between 25 and 30 means that you are overweight. A BMI over 30 tells us that someone is obese (very overweight).

It is possible to have a high BMI as a result of having lots of muscle, in which case the risks of stroke are not increased (unless you have built your muscles with the help of anabolic steroids!). It seems particularly harmful if much of your fat is around your middle. If, when you look down, you can't see your feet, you should definitely try to lose some weight.

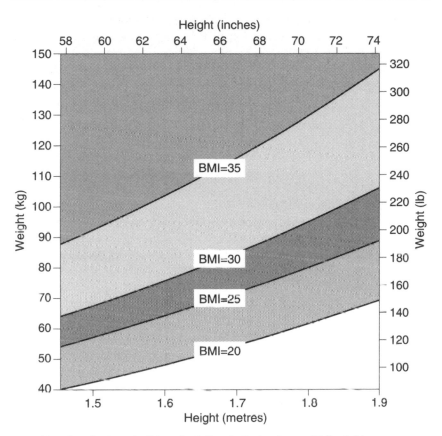

Use the chart or do this calculation to find out your BMI: divide your weight in kilograms by the square of your height in metres.

Your BMI score:
below 20: underweight
20–25: ideal
25–30: overweight
30+: seriously overweight – you need to see your doctor

Figure 6 The body mass index (BMI) chart

If your BMI is too high, especially if it's over 30, it is worth seeing a dietitian or your GP to get some sensible advice on diet and exercise. A BMI of less than 20 may mean that you are malnourished, especially if you have lost weight recently, and again it would be worth seeing your GP.

My cholesterol is normal. Does it really matter if I'm heavier than I should be?

Dieting is not just about getting your cholesterol down. Being overweight on its own is a 'risk factor' for stroke as well as for many other medical conditions such as osteoarthritis and gallstones. Being overweight will also make rehabilitation after your stroke more difficult. It takes more muscle strength to move a heavy body around than a light one. The risk of pressure sores and skin infections is also greater if you are overweight.

Because I'm overweight, I'm going to have to diet. How quickly should I lose weight?

Diets that result in very rapid weight loss are rarely of any value, because they are difficult to maintain and a few months later the weight has nearly always gone back on. Aim to make changes to your diet that you will be able to sustain, not just this week or month but for ever. That means switching to healthy but enjoyable eating in a way that reduces your total calorie intake a little. If you can lose one kilogram a month, in a year you will have lost 12 kilograms, and in two years' time you'll have a good excuse to get yourself a completely new set of clothes!

Is there anything that I should eat that will prevent me having another stroke?

'Antioxidants' may be of value in keeping the arteries healthy and possibly some other processes that happen with ageing, although so far they have not been shown in clinical trials to be beneficial. The theory is that they work by getting rid of 'free radicals', which are produced by normal chemical reactions in the body but can be harmful by, for example, helping cholesterol stick to the walls of your arteries.

Vitamins C and E are both effective antioxidants and can be found in fruit and vegetables and some vegetable oils. Some margarines are enriched with vitamin E. Green tea also has strong antioxidant properties. If you are eating a healthy diet containing plenty of fruit and vegetables, you will be getting adequate quantities of antioxidants. You can buy vitamin E capsules from health food shops if you wish to supplement your diet but there is nothing to be gained from exceeding a dose of 300mg per day. You can also supplement your diet with vitamin C but, so long as you are eating green vegetables and fresh fruit in adequate quantities (150–200g per day; five portions), it shouldn't really be necessary.

5
Speech and language

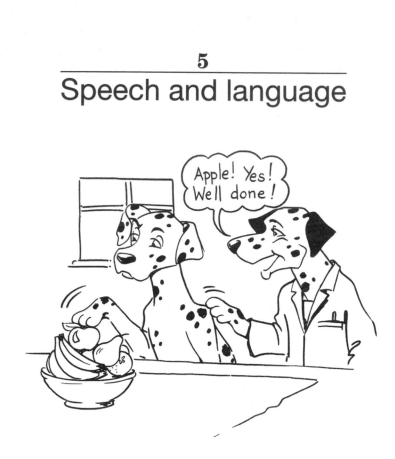

A stroke can affect a person's speech or language, or both. *Dysphasia* is a difficulty with language as a result of damage to the brain, and it can affect both speaking and writing. The problem can be a difficulty in understanding what is being said. This is called *receptive dysphasia*. It is a bit like suddenly being taken from Glasgow and deposited in the middle of Lithuania. You have no idea of what is being said to you, only with dysphasia it is even worse, because you probably won't even be able to make much sense of sign language either. Alternatively, the person may understand what is being said but be unable to find the right words to express what they want to say. This is called *expressive dysphasia*. We have all experienced the embarrassing situation of being introduced to someone, knowing perfectly well who they are and yet not being able to remember their name, or trying to remember something that is 'on the tip of our tongue'. Expressive dysphasia is like that, but for everything all the time. People often suffer from a mixture of both types.

Dysphasia most commonly occurs with strokes affecting the left side of the brain, so it often happens in a stroke survivor with paralysis of the right arm and leg. The only exception to this is in left-handed people, in about a third of whom their language area is on the right side of their brain.

Problems understanding and speaking

My son doesn't seem to understand anything I say to him, and talks nonsense. It's very worrying.

What you are describing is most likely to be due to dysphasia. His doctor or speech and language therapist will be able to tell you precisely what sort of dysphasia he has.

If you want to see whether he can understand you, ask him to do some simple actions that do not require him to respond verbally, such as closing his eyes or shaking your hand. If he can do that, see if he is able to point to some common objects such as a watch, a pen or a glass.

Dysphasia can easily be mistaken for confusion or a memory problem, and relatives are often worried that the person has suddenly become demented. With dysphasia the problem is solely with language. Although it is difficult to test them, because we need to use language to communicate, the other functions of the brain such as memory will be intact. Having dysphasia is incredibly frustrating. This is made worse by being treated as a halfwit or a child. Try to remember that the person is an adult and should be treated as one.

My husband can't understand speech and has great difficulty in saying anything. How can speech and language therapy help?

The speech and language therapist will start by identifying exactly what problems your husband has with his language. The descriptions of the types of dysphasia, given at the beginning of this chapter, are simple ones and a much more detailed examination and assessment is needed to plan a programme of treatment. Speech and language therapy can improve language by working on the impairments that are causing the dysphasia and teaching your husband strategies to get around some of the problems.

If possible, it would be worth your attending some of the therapy sessions to see what is being done and to find out the best way to communicate. There will also be exercises that you can work on between sessions.

Other problems

My husband came to England from Austria in 1939 and hasn't spoken German much since then. His English was perfect but since his stroke he talks only German, which I can't understand. What is going on?

When speech is lost as a result of stroke, what often remains is the first language learnt as a child. It is believed that, if two languages have been learnt at different times of life, they are stored in slightly different parts of the brain. So, if a bilingual person has a stroke, it is possible that only the part of the brain with one language in it is affected. This may be the case with your husband: the part where the English is stored has been affected but the part with German is intact. That he still has the German is a good sign that he will probably regain his other language skills eventually.

If possible, a bilingual speech and language therapist should be found to give him treatment; alternatively, if you have any friends or relatives who are fluent in both languages, it might be helpful if they could attend some of the therapy sessions to help him.

My wife sounds as if she is drunk when she speaks. She gets so embarrassed when friends visit that she doesn't even try to talk to them. What can be done to help her?

Where *dysphasia* is a difficulty with language generally, *dysarthria* is difficulty with speaking. Dysarthria can result from a stroke in any of several parts of the brain. It happens because of weakness of the muscles of the face, tongue or throat. Even if your wife's muscles are not weak, they may be stiff and this too can result in difficulty in speaking clearly (articulation). With some people their voice may also sound different. Dysarthria can occur with a stroke affecting the cerebellum – the part of the brain that helps co-ordinate the muscles. It can be made worse by problems not directly related to the stroke. For example, if your wife has poorly fitting dentures, a dry mouth or a sore tongue, these can also result in speech sounding slurred. Finding the real cause and getting the speech and language therapist to advise on treatment will usually help and eventually lead to improvement in your wife's clarity of speech.

A problem that sometimes goes unrecognised is a *dyspraxia* of the muscles controlling articulation. Dyspraxia is a difficulty in performing complex tasks consciously. Although each of the individual muscles seems to be working well when tested separately and there is no paralysis, they cannot work in the sequence required for tasks such as speaking or swallowing. So, for example, if you ask a person with dyspraxia to put their tongue out they may not be able to do it but they may be able to put their tongue out to lick their lips without thinking. With a dyspraxia of speech it may be very difficult to pronounce words clearly and sometimes people are unable to make any sound at all.

My brother can't get any words out, but when I took him to the carol service he sang the words to the hymns. Why is this?

When we learn music the information is stored on the right side of the brain in most people. This includes the words that go with the songs. So when someone becomes dysphasic because a stroke has affected the left side of the brain, the language that was learnt as part of music is preserved and still accessible. Unfortunately, the fact that your brother managed the words of the hymns does not necessarily mean that he is now beginning to recover his language.

I used to sing in a choir before I had my stroke, but now I just can't pitch the notes right. My speech wasn't affected, so why has this happened?

Music and some of the other artistic skills are based predominantly in the right side of brain (except in some left-handed people in whom everything is reversed). It is therefore likely that the stroke affected part of your right temporal lobe. What you are experiencing sounds very similar to a nun who came to my [AR] clinic: she woke one morning feeling perfectly well, made her way to mass – where she was responsible for leading the singing – and shocked her fellow nuns by the appalling noises she made. The only sign that she had had a stroke was her inability to sing. Over a period of a few months she recovered much of her former skill but was never quite trusted in the choir again.

A speech therapist with training in voice may be able to help you; otherwise, the best solution might be for you to go to a singing teacher and learn again from scratch.

My wife has recovered a little speech but sometimes she just gets stuck on one sound and keeps repeating it. It's really irritating. What can we do?

This is called *perseveration* and it occurs in some people with dysphasia. What happens is that the first word she says gets stuck in her memory circuits and keeps being repeated, regardless of whether it is still appropriate. For example, someone handing out the teas might ask: 'Do you want a cup of tea?' which is answered 'Yes'. 'Do you want milk in your tea?' 'Yes.' 'Do you want sugar in your tea?' 'Yes.' 'Do you want me to pour the tea over your head?' 'Yes.' . . . The fact is that she likes her tea black, without sugar and served at the table. Sometimes the perseveration is just for a sound rather than a whole word, but either way it is a difficult problem to manage. As soon as your wife starts repeating the sounds, try to stop her by distracting her with something else, because the longer it goes on the more difficult it is for her to break the habit. Leave plenty of time between questions so that her brain has time to clear before she is asked to respond again. For some people this can be as long as half a minute between questions.

Perseveration can also happen for movement, so that the person keeps on doing the same action repeatedly. Again the advice is the same: break up actions into small bits and take each stage slowly, allowing plenty of time and trying not to get impatient.

My brother is paralysed down the left-hand side. I was told that his speech wasn't affected but to me his voice seems different. And he hardly looks at me when he speaks.

This is a problem that happens frequently but is rarely recognised. Although language is usually controlled from the left side of the brain, music is generally controlled from the right side. As a result, the normal intonation and expression that we put into speech can be lost. The voice sounds flat and can be mistaken for depression. The fact that it is usually accompanied by difficulty in 'non-verbal communication' – facial expression and gesture – adds to the impression of someone who is miserable. As with the other problems, your brother will probably improve with time, patience and work. The speech and language therapist will be able to advise on the sort of exercises he should practise to speed recovery.

It is also possible that your brother is depressed. If you think that this is the case, tell the doctor. It is important to consider the possibility of depression, as it can be treated.

The voice can also be affected if there is slurring of speech due to weakness or poor control of the muscles that are used in speaking. This is called *dysarthria* and is described in an earlier answer.

Speech and language therapy

My husband is going to be given speech and language therapy. How much should he be getting and how long will it need to carry on for?

This will depend on the type and severity of the problem. The amount of therapy needed will also be affected by how much tolerance and concentration power your husband has. In the early days after a stroke people can often manage only a few minutes of therapy before they lose attention or need sleep. At this stage, frequent short sessions are best. Later, as his concentration improves, so can the length of the treatments. If your husband has a significant dysphasia that has developed within the last three months, he should probably have therapy at least three times a week for up to three months after it began. After that time it may be appropriate to continue at that sort of intensity or, if his progress is very slow, to reduce the frequency. The speech and language therapist should discuss any changes to therapy with you and your husband before they are made.

Language seems to improve at a different rate from that of some of the other impairments such as movement. It is slower to start showing improvement but carries on for longer – people sometimes continue to make progress two to three years after the stroke. Recovering from dysphasia is a long, laborious process. It is almost as frustrating for the carers as for the individual. The important thing is not to give up and to keep learning together. It can be very tempting to keep interpreting what your husband wants to say and to end up doing all the speaking for him because it is quicker and perhaps less embarrassing. Try not to do this, as it will not help him in his recovery. Confidence is half the battle, and this needs to be carefully nurtured.

Many areas have self-help groups for people with dysphasia where they and their carers can meet to socialise and help each other solve problems. Organisations such as Connect, The Stroke Association or Speakability (formerly Action for Dysphasic Adults or ADA) usually run these, and your speech and language therapist should have details of where and when they meet. Otherwise, contact their headquarters (addresses in Appendix 1) for information about groups near you.

How long will it take for my husband's speech to get back to normal?

This is a very hard question to answer, particularly in the first few weeks after a stroke. The scope for improvement depends on a lot of factors, including your husband's age, his motivation, the area affected by the stroke and how severe the stroke was. Also, every person is different, which makes it even more difficult to predict progress. The doctors and speech and language therapists are not being difficult when they tell you they don't know – they really don't!

After the first few weeks it is usually possible to give an idea of how slow or fast the recovery process may be, and also to judge from the progress already made whether it is realistic to think that things will return to normal. However, one of the most important factors is you and your husband working to improve things. People constantly surprise us.

My wife has dysphasia and can't talk. Would it help if I brought in my old typewriter?

It is very likely that if your wife has dysphasia she will also have problems with writing (*dysgraphia*), spelling and reading (*dyslexia*). All of the areas of the brain responsible for these tasks are very close together and depend on one another to function effectively. So it is unlikely that a typewriter will solve her problems with communication. She will probably have as much difficulty finding the right words whether she tries to say them or to write or type them. People with this problem often have difficulty even spelling their own name.

To begin with, try to get her to say 'Yes' and 'No' consistently. Ask questions that require only a 'yes' or 'no' answer, and give her plenty of time to reply. Her brain may be capable of under-standing the question and giving the correct answer but it may just be very slow. If you keep on bombarding her with questions or information, her brain will just become flooded with a mass of information, which will make her frustrated and angry. As she begins talking again, gradually increase the complexity of the information you give and help her to regain her vocabulary, in much the same way as one learns a foreign language. The speech and language therapist can give you advice about the best way to help. Constant repetition and hard work are really the only way to make progress.

We've seen catalogues showing expensive bits of equipment we can get to help my sister with her communication problems. Should we buy any?

No amount of sophisticated equipment will be able to compensate for a severe *dysphasia* – difficulty using language. Simple things, such as picture charts illustrating everyday needs such as food, drink, toilet and bed, can be tried, but even these may prove difficult to use if your sister has severe difficulty with understanding. Computer programs have been used with some success in retraining language but there is no guarantee.

If her problem is one of difficulty in articulation due to *dysarthria* (difficulty in speaking) or *dyspraxia* (difficulty in doing complex tasks) but without a problem with language, communication aids can be tremendously helpful. Simple keyboards or computers can be used, although a pen and paper are often easier. The speech and language therapist will help to advise what is most suitable for your sister. More sophisticated electronics can generate the sounds of words typed onto a keyboard or can be pre-programmed to say different things at the touch of a specific button.

We know of two computer programs for speech: INTACT, produced by the Frenchay Hospital in Bristol, and REACT, produced by the Speech and Language Therapy Department of the Borders Health Authority (addresses in Appendix 1). King's College Hospital in London has an Assistive Technology Team offering a co-ordinated approach to assessment of assistive technology (e.g. environmental controls, computers, communication aids, powered wheelchairs). The team includes therapists, a doctor and a rehabilitation engineer. Assessments are done at home or in the centre. For more information, contact Kings Healthcare (details in Appendix 1).

There are probably other similar centres around the country, so ask your doctor if there is anything in your area.

6
Personal care

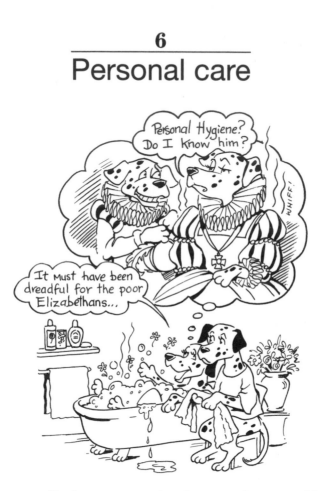

A stroke can affect many aspects of personal care and hygiene. Apart from making it difficult to use the toilet, there can be incontinence of urine (wetting oneself) or of faeces (messing oneself), or both. This can be very distressing both to the individual and to their family but there are solutions. The important thing is to find out why it is happening and get expert advice on how best to deal with the problem.

Incontinence

My mother was always such a private person and so clean. Now she just wets herself and can't even control her bowels, and it really upsets her.

This may be the result of several things. Sometimes the area of the brain that controls the bladder and the bowels has been damaged, so the person has no control over these functions. However, there could be other reasons, so anyone suffering from incontinence longer than four weeks after a stroke should have several tests; this may mean some investigations of the bladder and bowels and how they work. When the cause of the problem is diagnosed, the right way to manage it can be worked out.

It is important to remember that your mother is not doing this deliberately and is probably very depressed about it – which can make the problem worse. By getting expert advice and help in dealing with the problem, you may well find that she starts to improve and take an active part in getting back to a more normal life, and being her old self.

Since my wife had a stroke, she keeps wetting herself. Why is this, and what can be done about it?

A stroke sometimes affects the part of the brain that controls the urge to urinate (pass water), so ordinary 'voluntary' control is lost. In most – but not all – people this improves as the brain heals, and continence is usually regained by three months after the stroke. If your wife has had this difficulty for more than a month, it may be due to a problem with her bladder, so she should be properly assessed by a urologist (a doctor who specialises in bladder and urinary problems). This should help find out the precise cause of her problem.

If your wife's incontinence is related to her stroke and nothing else, the doctors and nurses should arrange for you to have advice from a nurse specialist continence adviser, who can help you find the best way to deal with the problem at home. (If you like, you can contact the Continence Foundation – details in Appendix 1 – to find an adviser near you.) There is no reason why – with the right advice and equipment – it cannot be managed conveniently, comfortably and hygienically.

They put a catheter into my husband's waterworks immediately he arrived in casualty, and it's been there ever since. Is he going to need it forever?

It rather depends on why he had the catheter (tube) put in. Sometimes a urinary catheter is used to deal with incontinence after a stroke. This may be necessary if your husband's skin is very fragile and might become easily damaged by contact with the chemicals in his urine. The other reason why a catheter may be used in the casualty department is that your husband was unable to pass urine on his own and his bladder had become painfully swollen. This is called *retention of urine*, and is best treated by inserting a catheter to let the urine out. Later on the doctor will investigate to find out why it has happened. In men the most common reason is an enlarged prostate gland, although there are other reasons such as being very constipated.

Once the main reason for the catheter being put in has passed, there should be a period when your husband tries to do without it. If a catheter is left in for a long time there is a danger that, by keeping the bladder empty all the time, the bladder can lose its ability to contract and work normally. If this were to happen with your husband, when the catheter was suddenly removed he would find that he could not control his passing of urine. To prevent this, some days before the catheter is to be removed the staff may clamp it for a few hours at a time, gradually increasing the time between releasing it and thus allowing his bladder to regain some of its normal 'tone'. However, if the catheter is left in for too long without any attempt to retrain his bladder, it will be more difficult for him to manage without it. So talk to the staff about your worry.

There are different products around to enable people to do without a catheter despite their incontinence. For men there are adapted sheaths that can be worn over the penis all the time to channel the flow of urine into a container. The hospital staff (or the GP and district nurse, if you are at home) should advise about the best type to use and how to get hold of them locally. It will be important to ensure that the sheath is changed regularly and his genital area kept clean to prevent infection. The sheath can be difficult to use for some men, particularly if their penis is small.

Is there any equipment that my wife can use to help with her incontinence?

Catheters and incontinence pads are the same for men and women, although catheters for women are shorter. No one has yet designed a sheath suitable for women. The other difficulty is finding the equivalent of a man's urinal or bottle that can be used easily by women while sitting in a chair or lying in bed. There are some so-called slipper pans that slide under the bottom and are used effectively by some people. But your wife needs to be able to lift her bottom at least a little way off the chair and to have good hand function at least on one side. It is also very easy to spill the contents of the pan, so it is not exactly an ideal solution. Given that 10–20% of women of retirement age are incontinent of urine either regularly or occasionally, there is a huge undeveloped market for an effective way of managing the problem.

If my husband doesn't recover control over his bladder, what can we do? I wouldn't be able to cope with him wetting all the time.

If he remains incontinent, there are several ways to deal with it. It will be very important for you and your husband to receive expert advice. Your hospital will probably have a nurse continence adviser who can make sure that your husband has the right equipment and support to go home. If you are unsure of what is available in your area, contact the Continence Foundation (see Appendix 1). They run a telephone helpline, staffed by continence nurse advisers who have a database of all local continence services, so could advise you of the ones in your area.

Before your husband comes home you should both be given advice on the most appropriate methods to deal with any incontinence, and be put in touch with the local support services such as laundry services and equipment delivery. There are many excellent products to help people deal with urinary incontinence, which can be supplied direct to your home on a regular basis by your local services.

Not being able to control my bladder is one of the worst things about the stroke – I hardly dare leave the house. But nothing seems to have been done about it. Is there any way it can be cured?

Many people overcome their incontinence after a stroke by training their bladder to work normally. This is a bit like fitness training. You need to be quite disciplined and go to the toilet at regular intervals – initially every two hours. This means that your bladder never really fills up and takes control. You keep the control and your bladder learns to empty itself at your command. You will be surprised how quickly you find an improvement – even after only a couple of weeks you will be able to increase the time between visits to the toilet.

To allow yourself some sleep at night you should continue to wear the incontinence pads. If you make sure you empty your bladder before you settle for the night and then wake yourself early to do the same again, things should gradually start to improve for the night as well.

Sometimes a urinary infection can really upset all plans for training your bladder. In this situation you may find that you are unable to last for even two hours before passing urine. The reason for this is that the infection in the urine makes your bladder very irritable and more difficult to control. With an infection you will also notice that your urine has an unpleasant fishy smell. You should see your doctor straight away, and he or she will take a specimen of your urine before starting you on a course of antibiotics. You should notice a big improvement in everything once the infection is cured.

Are there any drugs available to help with my incontinence?

It depends on the underlying cause of your incontinence. One of the common causes after a stroke is what is called an unstable bladder. This is where the bladder starts contracting and emptying when it is only partly full. If this is the case for you, there are drugs that do sometimes work. The most widely used of these are oxybutynin and tolterodine, which can sometimes be dramatically effective.

The other drug that can help is called DDAVP (or desmopressin). This is a manufactured version of antidiuretic hormone, which the body produces normally to regulate the amount of urine the kidneys make. The DDAVP is taken as a spray up the nose, and its effect is to reduce the amount of urine produced for a few hours afterwards. It is most useful for people who find that they wet the bed at night. A sniff of the drug just before going to sleep often results in a dry night. It is also good to take it before long journey or when you know that it is going to be difficult to change your pad or use a toilet.

I keep getting infections in my urine. Are they related to my recent stroke? If so, how can I prevent them?

Urinary infections may occur more frequently in people who are not able to move about very much, because this can encourage a condition in which the bladder does not empty properly when they pass urine. The urine left behind can become infected because there is time for any bacteria present in it to multiply and then set up an infection in the bladder wall. Once this happens, an infection is very hard to shift because a little bit probably stays behind all the time, even after a course of antibiotics. When you are being treated for an infection, it may help to drink plenty of water, so the bacteria keep getting flushed away.

To get over the problem of some urine remaining in the bladder when you use the toilet, it is sometimes helpful to try to pass urine again after the first stream has ended. If, at the same time, you press on the bladder (the area just above the pubic bone at the lower end of your abdomen), you will often find that a bit more urine comes out. This will stop any bacteria having the chance to grow in the urine if it stayed in your bladder. Along with these methods it is very important to be particular about your own personal hygiene to prevent any infection passing up from the genital area into your bladder.

Drinking a glass or two of cranberry juice every day can sometimes help to prevent urine infections. It's not clear precisely what the juice does but it has been suggested that something in the cranberry juice stops the bacteria from attaching themselves to the wall of the bladder. Cranberry juice is quite easy to get hold of – it can be bought in most supermarkets and chemist/pharmacist shops, and actually tastes quite nice.

Since the stroke I keep 'messing' myself. There just doesn't seem to be anything I can do to control my bowels. I feel so ashamed and disgusting having to be cleaned up by the nurses. What can I do?

Becoming *incontinent of faeces* after a stroke is common, occurring in about a quarter of stroke survivors. It can result from the stroke affecting the part of the brain involved in controlling bowel movements and, in most such cases, as the rest of the body improves so does the bowel control. It can also result from becoming constipated! If your rectum becomes full of faeces that you can't get rid of, the more liquid faeces higher up the bowel can squeeze past the solid faeces and escape through the anus (the opening from the bowel) that is stretched open by the constipated faeces. If this is the case for you, enemas and laxatives will eventually solve the problem. It may take several enemas to put things completely right. Other causes of faecal incontinence are too much laxative and infections in the bowel causing diarrhoea. Your doctor may need to take a sample of your faeces to check that you don't have an infection.

Even if your incontinence can't be cured, it is nearly always possible to control it so that you don't open your bowels at unexpected times. This involves giving you a drug such as codeine or loperamide to cause the stool to be more solid, and then giving you regular enemas, either daily or every second day, to keep your rectum empty.

You are not alone in the world, having incontinence of faeces. A recent study of people living at home (not stroke patients) found that 11% of men and 15% of women over the age of 50 years had the problem.

Constipation

I've got really constipated. What treatments are there?

The best treatment for constipation is to try to prevent it by eating plenty of fruit and vegetables and other foods that are high in fibre. It is also important to drink plenty each day (about eight glasses of fluid). However, if this does not work, you may need to take a regular laxative. Discuss with your doctor what type would be best for you. The problem with laxatives is that your bowel becomes accustomed to them, which can lead to your needing higher and higher doses for them to work properly. Another disadvantage of laxatives is that they can cause your intestines (gut) to contract very strongly, which can be painful.

Laxatives work in two ways. In one they stimulate the bowel to contract, forcing the faeces through more effectively; senna (Senokot) works in this way. There are also more powerful stimulants, which your doctor can prescribe if necessary. The other type of laxative softens the faeces; lactulose is the most commonly used of this sort. A problem with lactulose is that it causes a lot of gas (wind) to be formed in the bowel which, if you cannot move about, may be difficult to get rid of and will make you feel bloated and uncomfortable. The macrogol Movicol is a powder that needs to be dissolved in water before being drunk; it can be very effective and is becoming one of the most favoured laxatives. Co-danthramer is also occasionally prescribed; it works by both stimulating the bowel and softening the faeces, but can cause a painful rash around your bottom.

Other methods of dealing with constipation include

suppositories and enemas, both of which are placed in your back passage (rectum). This may seem rather extreme but in some parts of Europe suppositories are a very common way of taking various forms of medicine. Suppositories are small capsules containing a substance that will gently encourage the lower bowel to work within half an hour. A nurse can give these to you very easily and could teach you to do it yourself. Enemas are rather stronger than suppositories. They are usually used if you have been constipated for some time and there is an immovable block of hard faeces in your rectum, and suppositories have not worked. These days enemas come in specially prepared kits that contain about half a cupful of a substance similar to soapy water (which was the treatment used in the old days when much larger amounts were given through a funnel and tubing!). Again, a nurse can give you this and show you or your relative how to administer it yourselves at home.

Sometimes constipation is so bad that none of these things will work and then a nurse or doctor will need to remove the faeces stuck in the lower back passage by hand. Whatever the cause of your constipation, it is important for your comfort not to let things get too bad, because the early treatments are relatively simple and easy to use. You should consult your doctor if you have continuing problems with constipation, to make sure you are using the most effective method of dealing with it.

Skin care

I often get sore skin beneath my breasts and in the groin. How can this be prevented?

Sore skin under the breasts and in the groin occurs as a result of sweating between the skin surfaces in these areas. Sometimes this is made worse in the groin by the effects of incontinence of urine and/or faeces. Whatever the cause, the skin can break down and sometimes the area becomes very sore. It can also easily become infected with the infection thrush.

The best way to prevent the skin from breaking down and getting infected is to try to keep these areas as clean and dry as possible, and to wear cotton underwear (which will absorb the sweat). If you do not wear a bra, use some form of cotton padding (even a folded cotton handkerchief) between your breasts and the skin they rest on, to absorb the sweat and help keep skin surfaces apart. Washing the areas twice a day, or regular bathing, is essential. If the soreness is aggravated by thrush, your doctor will be able to recommend a special anti-fungal cream such as clotrimazole (Canesten) to rub in.

If the soreness in your groin is linked with problems of leaking urine, it is important to talk to your doctor or nurse about it. There are plenty of good pads they can suggest, which, like babies' disposable nappies, protect your skin and keep your groin area dry and comfortable.

The nurses say it's important not to let my father develop pressure sores. What are they, and why do people get them?

Pressure sores are the result of people lying in bed in the same position for too long on a hard surface. The skin against the hard surface (even a mattress) gets pressed against the bone underneath it and the blood flow to that area gradually gets cut off, causing the skin to die. This is most common in people who are very ill and unable to move themselves in bed, and who are also malnourished and thin. The problem can happen in susceptible people over just a few hours. Sometimes there is just a reddening of the skin where the pressure was greatest, but when the area is badly affected it becomes black as it dies and a sore develops – which can cover an area as wide and as deep as a fist. If a pressure sore is very deep, it may go down as far as the bone; this is serious, because it can lead to infection in the bone, which is very hard to treat and can even be fatal. It is also extremely painful.

If your father were to develop pressure sores, they would take a long time to heal. They require special dressings by a nurse or doctor. Sometimes the wound created has to be cleaned and specially dressed in an operating theatre. It is for all these reasons that doctors and nurses take pressure sores very seriously indeed.

The best action is to prevent them from occurring in the first place. When people are admitted to hospital after a stroke, they are usually assessed for the likely risk of their developing pressure sores so that the right preventive action can be included as part of their care. When they are discharged home, similar precautions should be in place if the person is still regarded as being at particular risk.

There are many products that are used to prevent pressure sores. These include:

- small items (e.g. fleece bootees or pads) for particularly bony parts of the body such as the ankles and elbows, which are particularly at risk in some people,

- cushions specially made to even out the pressure when someone is sitting,

- special mattresses and beds that protect the whole body from having pressure being too strong at any one point.

You may also have noticed that the staff regularly change your father's position in bed, because he cannot yet move himself. This is to prevent his having pressure for too long on any particular part of his body.

My husband is coming home soon but I am frightened that he will get pressure sores like my neighbour's husband did. How do they happen and is there anything I can do to prevent them?

Sometimes people get pressure sores when they are at home because they are unable to move themselves. The staff in the hospital should assess your home before your husband is discharged, to make sure that he will be able to cope . . . with your help. They can then make sure that you are provided with the necessary equipment to keep him safe and comfortable. Because lying (or sitting) in the same position for too long can cause pressure sores, you may also need advice and training on how to move him without injuring yourself. You may need special equipment to help you so that you do not strain your back, and this can be arranged for you by the hospital staff in conjunction with your local authority's social services department.

What should I do if my wife gets a pressure sore?

If she gets a pressure sore at home, it should be reported to her doctor as soon as possible, so that arrangements can be made for the appropriate treatment and help for you. Special mattresses and cushions are available for people to use at home, just as in hospital. A very important factor in causing pressure sores is poor nutrition, and you should see if you can persuade her to eat more. If necessary, get some of the energy- and protein-rich food supplements such as Entera or Fresubin from her doctor.

My partner has developed a pressure sore and it's causing him a lot of pain. What can be done to make him more comfortable?

Pressure sores can be very sore indeed, and unfortunately there are no magic answers to dealing with your partner's. The first thing is to make sure it is healing. All the measures described in the answers to the earlier questions should be used, such as the special mattress and the dressings to the wound. He will be more comfortable if he doesn't lie on the sore. He may well get relief from simple pain-killers such as paracetamol taken regularly, but may require something stronger if these don't work – which would need to be prescribed for him by the doctor.

7
Memory, mood and sleep

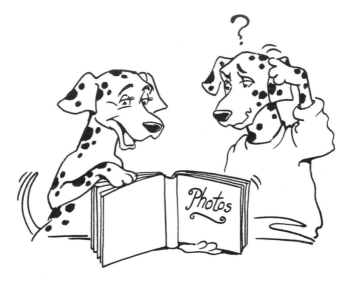

A single stroke can, and in most cases will, affect some aspects of brain function, such as use of language – understanding, finding the right words and speaking – understanding abstract thinking, using arithmetic, writing, recognising objects and identifying familiar faces. People can have problems understanding time and place, and many other intellectual processes.

Unlike dementia, stroke will not affect all of these processes and they will not get progressively worse. Memory can be affected if the temporal lobe is involved in the stroke. Personality may change if the front part of the brain is damaged. However, as with other aspects of a person's stroke, these functions may well improve over time and with practice.

It is not uncommon for stroke survivors to become depressed. This is a natural reaction to the significant impact the illness will have on their lives but it is important to be alert to the possibility of severe depression, which can be treated.

Memory

My partner has been confused since having the stroke. Will he get better or does he have dementia now?

If he was not confused before the stroke, he does not have dementia now. The definition of dementia is 'a progressive condition that has been developing for at least three months'. The two most common causes are Alzheimer's disease and multiple small strokes (called multi-infarct dementia). You mention that your partner has had only one stroke, so it is unlikely that he has dementia now. A single stroke can often affect some of the 'thinking' aspects of a person's brain. Unlike dementia, though, it will not affect all of them and will not keep getting worse.

The psychologist came to see my wife, but she's not mad – she has just had a stroke. What was the psychologist doing?

A psychologist is not the same as a psychiatrist, although their work does overlap in some respects. Unfortunately, only a small proportion of hospitals treating stroke patients have access to psychologists, whose particular expertise is in recognising and treating problems with memory, personality and perception (awareness of and understanding one's environment). Some of these difficulties will be obvious; others will only be spotted after formal testing and yet may have an important impact on recovery, particularly of higher level function such as getting back to work or regaining special skills that your wife worked hard to get earlier on in life. There are many occasions when a psychological assessment helps to identify why someone is having unexpected difficulty with some aspects of rehabilitation. Having found where the problem is, it may then be possible to devise new ways of doing things to get around it.

An assessment by a psychologist usually involves a series of tests of memory, language, numeracy and perception that many people will have done before in the form of intelligence tests. They will include some measures to evaluate the level that your wife would have been performing at before the stroke. Because the tests require a lot of concentration, it is usually necessary to spread them over several sessions. Having identified the areas that have been affected by the stroke, the psychologist will then work in collaboration with the other members of the team to devise the most appropriate rehabilitation programme.

Some psychologists also work with physicians and psychiatrists to help treat 'mood disturbance', such as depression or anxiety. They may have counselling skills that are of use in helping the stroke survivor and their carer come to terms with the effects of the illness. Later on, when your wife might want to go back to work or resume previous activities and interests, the psychologist will be able to advise on what changes might be necessary and how best to achieve them.

My memory just isn't what it was. Is that due to the stroke, and will it recover?

There are three reasons why your memory may seem worse following your stroke.

First, the stroke has caused damage to nerve cells, so it is not surprising that your memory is affected to some extent. Memory can recover but, even if it doesn't, it is possible to learn to use what is left more effectively. Working out ways to overcome memory problems is something that many of us find we have to do as we get older, and is not a problem solely for people after stroke. Making more effort to remember the important things, consigning the trivial things to the mental dustbin, writing things down and using the memories of the people around you are all ways to get round the problem. It is common for particular areas of memory to be affected more severely than others. For example, you may find it difficult to recognise faces or recall their names, even for people you know well. This can be very embarrassing, particularly if you have only just been introduced to someone. Sometimes people repeat the name frequently when talking to them, especially at the beginning. Americans often seem to do this. 'It's really good to meet you, Mrs Smith. Tell me, Mrs Smith, have you been here long? Do you know many people here, Mrs Smith?' And so on.

Secondly, a stroke can affect your ability to concentrate, which will affect how much you remember. This is likely to be a particular problem in the first few months after the stroke, when you may well be feeling tired all the time – you are having to learn all sorts of new things, you will have met a lot of new people and things around you feel strange. The problem with concentration will be made worse by worrying that you are losing your memory and developing dementia. As with many of the other effects of stroke, it is a question of giving yourself time to recover, not becoming totally preoccupied with it and yet at the same time exercising your brain to improve your concentration. A mistake that people often make is to attribute every single problem to the

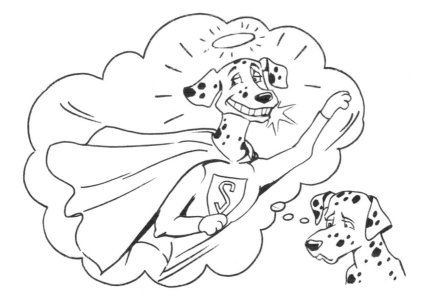

stroke. It is unlikely that you were perfect before the stroke, yet it is only when you have had a major illness that you start looking at yourself in a critical way. Try not to become too introspective, because it will affect your ability to recover. It will take a lot of courage to force yourself back into situations where your memory and ability to concentrate are tested. Judging the right time to go back to work, for example, could be difficult and it would be worth discussing this subject with your doctor, employer and perhaps the company doctor.

One way of building up your memory and concentration skills is to listen to a radio or television programme and take notes. Or read a passage from a book and then write down the key points. You can gradually increase the length of the passage and the difficulty of the subject matter but don't expect to be as quick or as fluent initially as you think you used to be.

A third reason why your memory may not seem to be as good as before is if you have developed some depression. Even mild mood disturbance can affect your ability to concentrate and remember things. Severe depression, which is quite common after stroke, can manifest itself as profound memory loss. If you do have severe depression, it is very important to make sure that this is diagnosed, as treatment can be highly effective.

Mood

My husband is just so miserable all the time. The doctors say it's not surprising given the severity of his stroke, but that doesn't help him or me!

The doctors are right when they say that it is not surprising that he feels miserable. About four out of every ten people develop significant depression after their stroke. There are two explanations for this. The obvious one is that he has suffered a major loss very similar to a bereavement. He has lost a lot of independence. He may have lost his job, his status and often the respect of his friends and colleagues. Plans that you and he might have made for the future will probably need to be rethought. The relationship between him and the rest of the family, including you, may have suddenly changed, which can have affected him deeply. Given these possible changes, it is perhaps surprising that more people don't become depressed.

It is also possible that the effect of the stroke on your husband's brain has produced mood disturbance regardless of how severe his disability is. There may be centres in the brain that control how we feel, and if they are damaged then depression will result.

The first thing to be done is to make sure that your husband *is* depressed and that there is not some other explanation.

- If he is in pain, this should be treated, as pain can cause great misery.

- Is he unhappy because he doesn't understand what is happening to him? Sometimes giving clearer explanations, allowing him to express what is worrying him and helping him to regain some control over his life will be enough to help lift his mood.

- If his stroke has resulted from damage to the right or 'non-dominant' side of his brain, he may have lost some of his ability to show emotion through facial expression and tone of voice, and this can sometimes be misinterpreted as depression.

The classic symptoms of depression include feeling as if everything is pointless and worthless, having low self-esteem, having little or no interest in the things going on, poor appetite and disturbed sleep. This last can either be difficulty in getting off to sleep or waking in the early hours of the morning and being unable to get back to sleep, usually lying awake worrying. Mornings are usually the worst times for people with depression. Going to bed, hoping they don't wake up in the morning and considering how they might end their life are symptoms of serious depression and need urgent attention.

You will be particularly aware of his change in personality. It can be very frustrating trying to inject some interest into his life and not getting any response. He is likely to lose interest in you sexually, and if he does try he may well be unable to perform. This may only increase his sense of worthlessness. He may cry at the least provocation or become angry and withdrawn. All this can be terribly hard on you and can put a serious strain on your relationship just when it is important to support each other. Depression should be regarded as an infectious disease – it is quite common to see it happening in both partners.

My wife has been very depressed after her stroke. Is there any treatment available for her?

If you think depression is a possibility, seek help from her doctors. The answer might be for her to discuss her problem with an expert who can provide guidance and support. Alternatively, medicines may be considered. Antidepressants can be very effective, with no (or only minor) side effects. There are many different drugs that can be used and your doctor will try to choose one most appropriate for your wife. The older drugs mainly belong to the group called the tricyclic antidepressants. Examples are amitriptyline, imipramine, lofepramine, nortriptyline and maprotiline. The possible unwanted effects are drowsiness, confusion, dry mouth and, in men, difficulty passing urine (passing water).

A newer group of drugs are the 'selective serotonin re-uptake inhibitors' (SSRIs). Among these are fluoxetine (Prozac), paroxetine and sertraline. They have fewer side effects so it is common to start with one of these. They tend to stimulate rather than sedate, so are usually taken in the morning, unlike the tricyclic antidepressants, which are usually given at bedtime. They can, unfortunately, sometimes damp down the person's appetite and this needs to looked out for.

Any drug might cause side effects, but it is impossible to predict what or in whom. If a problem does develop, it can usually be resolved within a day or two of stopping the drug. Nevertheless, all these drugs are powerful and should be used only under a doctor's supervision. All the antidepressants take at least two weeks, and sometimes as much as four or even six weeks, before they begin to start working. So try not to give up on them until they have had a chance to produce an effect. If one drug doesn't work or causes an unacceptable side effect, there are plenty of others to choose from. Your wife should probably take the drug for at least three to six months before stopping it; otherwise, there is a good chance that her depression will return. None of the drugs we've mentioned is addictive, so there won't be any problems when your wife stops taking it. If the depression returns after your wife has taken the drug for three months, her doctor will probably advise that she starts taking it again and then continuing to take it long term.

Very occasionally, if someone's depression is very severe indeed and it hasn't responded to drug treatment, the psychiatrist may advise electro-convulsive therapy (ECT). This has had a very bad press, not helped by the portrayal of it in the film *One Flew over the Cuckoo's Nest*. In fact, it can be life saving in certain circumstances. It is given under general anaesthetic and so does not cause any distress. ECT is not often used in the immediate aftermath of a stroke as the risks of making it worse are too great, but if severe depression is still present after three months, it might be considered.

Depression is a disease that people sometimes try to hide, thinking that it indicates they are weak and unable to deal with the stroke. This is clearly not the case. It can happen to anyone, however robust their personality. The earlier it is brought to the attention of the doctors, the easier it will be to treat. Don't ignore it, hoping it will just disappear.

I think my son is depressed but it is so difficult to tell because he can't talk.

It is difficult to diagnose depression when people are unable to express their thoughts and feelings. If your son has lost his ability to speak as a result of the stroke, doctors have to depend on watching his behaviour and facial expressions to make the diagnosis. His family and friends are likely to be better than the health professionals at identifying changes, so if you feel that depression is possible, don't hesitate to tell the doctors. Often the best way of confirming this is by starting treatment with an antidepressant and looking to see if there is improvement. The newer drugs are so safe that this is a perfectly reasonable strategy to adopt.

Sometimes my husband just bursts into tears without warning and at the slightest provocation. What am I doing wrong?

You are doing nothing wrong. Stroke can cause what is called *emotional lability* or *emotionalism*. People affected by this will cry or, less commonly, laugh for little or no reason. Sometimes they will switch rapidly from one to the other. We all have differing degrees of control over our emotions: men are usually taught early on that it is socially unacceptable to cry in public but this is not usually the case with women. Biologically, there is no reason why there should be a difference between the sexes – it is simply a difference in what our society or culture sees as 'normal'. The emotions are sometimes very close to the surface after a stroke and are no longer under the same degree of voluntary control that they used to be.

You will probably find that your husband is more likely to start crying when he hears about things related to him, his family or home than by subjects not so closely related to his own life. This problem will be more severe if there is also an element of depression but can certainly exist even if he is not depressed. He might say that he doesn't know why he is crying, as he doesn't feel unhappy. It is a distressing symptom both for him and for you. Usually it settles as the stroke recovers. Treatment with fluoxetine (Prozac) can help, the benefits being evident within a few days – which is much quicker than when the drug is being used to treat depression.

Try not to be embarrassed by the crying, and avoid the temptation to keep all communication with him at such a bland level that the symptom is avoided. In the long run, that might only delay his ability to recover control over his emotions.

He's not the same person I married. He used to have such a fiery temper and now he just doesn't seem to care about anything.

If depression is part of your husband's 'post-stroke phase', he should be given treatment for this, as low dosage antidepressants can be very effective in helping to lift the depression. Some stroke and rehabilitation units have psychologists attached to them, and it may be helpful to see one together for a number of sessions for advice and assistance. The psychologist may also be able to give your husband some help with any memory and concentration problems.

My son seems to be having hallucinations – seeing things that aren't there and saying the nurses have been doing things to him that I know are not true. Why is this?

Damage to certain parts of his brain from the stroke can have resulted in hallucinations – imagining things that aren't really there – or misinterpretation of what is going on around him. Hallucinations can seem very real to the person having them and it will probably be difficult to persuade your son that he is only imagining them.

After stroke, hallucinations are usually confined to seeing things (animals or people) but may sometimes involve hearing voices. Both sorts can be very distressing and sometimes frightening. Reassurance may be all that your son needs. If they occur only when it is dark, it may help to keep his light on. Sometimes it is necessary to give tranquillising drugs. In most cases the hallucinations will gradually go away and it shouldn't be necessary to continue on drugs for long.

Damage to the parietal lobe, particularly on the right side of the brain, can result in people having difficulties in recognising objects or even parts of their own body. This can lead to very strange thoughts and beliefs. For example, people can sometimes seem to totally ignore or 'disown' the whole of the left side of their body. This can lead to the situation where they no longer attempt, for example, to dress their left side or wash/shave the left side of their face. I [AR] had a patient who called me over one morning, picked up his left arm and said 'Look what my wife left behind last night'. Unable to identify his left arm as belonging to him, the only rational explanation he could find was that the last person to see him had left their arm behind. Another person complained that the nurse had got into bed with him the previous night. He had 'disowned' his left side and although he was vaguely aware of something being there, his conclusion was that it must have been one of the staff. In these two cases, although the sensation never completely returned to normal, it did recover sufficiently to stop the misinterpretations.

In both instances the complaints were clearly misunderstandings of reality, but there are sometimes situations where it is difficult to know what is true and what isn't. Always take seriously what your son says. Consider that a complaint might be genuine. Strange things can occur in hospital, and there can be little more distressing than being disbelieved when something really did happen.

Sleep

Ever since the stroke, my wife has complained of feeling tired, and she spends much of the day asleep. Why is this, and will she get better?

Tiredness is one of the most common complaints after a stroke and one that is often ignored by the health professionals. In the first few days after a stroke people frequently sleep all day, waking only when spoken to or receiving nursing care. This is probably due to brain swelling, which increases the pressure inside the head and causes a reduction in overall brain function.

There is little to be gained by trying to force your wife to stay awake for long periods. The best strategy is to wake her for short periods, perhaps at mealtimes, and then let her sleep. She will gradually increase the time she is alert, as the brain swelling subsides, but this may take several weeks, depending on the size and cause of her stroke. Even when this short-term problem settles, though, she is likely to feel drained and lacking in energy, possibly for many months. We don't know why this happens or the best treatment for it. It is possible that her normal day/night sleep pattern is disturbed and that the quality of sleep your wife is getting is less good. It makes sense to try to get her into the habit of being as active as possible during the day and really resist the temptation to cat nap. Any sleep she takes during the day will reduce the amount that she can achieve at night.

Trying to regain as much physical fitness as possible will also help. The time spent lying immobile in bed or recovering slowly from the effects of the stroke will have taken a toll on her heart, lung and muscle function. She will need to start rebuilding fitness from scratch, just as an athlete has to after an injury. An exercise programme should make her feel much better, with more energy, and may even help her regain some of the function she thought she had lost as a result of the stroke.

Persistent tiredness can be a symptom of depression, and this should be considered by her doctors. It is also worth reviewing what drugs she is taking and whether they are really needed. Some antidepressants, some pain-killers, some of the drugs used to control muscle stiffness and all sleeping tablets can make people feel tired and lacking in energy.

I find it really difficult to sleep on the ward. Would it be all right to have sleeping tablets?

You should avoid taking sleeping tablets if at all possible. They all have side effects, you can become addicted to most of them and in the vast majority of cases they aren't necessary for your health. They all work by reducing brain activity, which is exactly the opposite of what you are trying to do in recovering from your stroke. Although they may increase the amount of sleep you get at night, you will pay the price of a hangover effect the next day and will be more likely to fall than someone who is not taking them. Moreover, when you stop taking them there could well be a period of several days or weeks when you feel agitated with very disturbed sleep patterns.

There is a saying that you can borrow sleep but you can't buy it; this neatly summarises the problem of getting onto sleeping tablets. It is very unusual for your body to deprive itself of sleep. You will need a certain amount of sleep each day – which will be less than usual if you are less active than usual. Any time you spend in a siesta or a cat nap in the daytime will shorten the amount you get at night. Although you might think you are not sleeping at all, you will be – even if it is just in short bursts with long gaps in between.

The first thing to do is try to establish why you are having difficulty sleeping:

- It can be difficult to get to sleep in a noisy ward.

- You probably won't be used to sleeping surrounded by other people.

- The bed will be strange and often harder than you are used to at home.

- You are likely to be anxious about yourself and your family.

- You may have some discomfort or pain, not least from any difficulty you have in moving yourself around the bed.

- You may find that you need to urinate more frequently at night than you are used to.

All these factors are good reasons for disturbed nights. If it is the noise, you will probably get used to it quite quickly. If not, it might be possible to be transferred to a single room – although there could be good reasons why this is not desirable, such as the nurses needing to keep a close eye on you. If you are in pain, the answer is to find the cause and reduce it or else take a pain-killer before going to bed. If your muscles are painful because you cannot change position, you may need a different sort of mattress or else the nurses should help you change position more frequently.

Sometimes a hot milky drink before going to sleep can help. If your doctors have no objection, a small alcoholic drink is a lot safer than a sleeping tablet and much more enjoyable! Forcing yourself to stay awake during the day and keeping your mind and body as active as possible will lead to more satisfying sleep. As a last resort, take a sleeping tablet but try not to indulge the temptation every night and certainly don't continue to take them when you get home.

If you were already taking sleeping tablets when you came into hospital, you will need to continue with them, as stopping them suddenly could make you unwell. However, use the opportunity of being in hospital to gradually reduce the dose, with the intention of doing without them altogether.

8

Pain and sensation

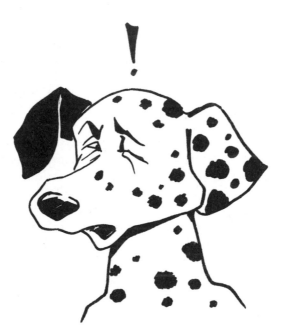

After a stroke, sensations are often misinterpreted by the skin: a light touch may feel like a burn and heat may feel cold. The problem is due to the brain misunderstanding the signals sent to it by the sensors in the skin and is not due to problems in the trunk or limbs themselves.

Pain

I have terrible pain down my right side. My stroke three months ago initially just caused mild weakness on the right, which recovered really well. Have I had another stroke, and what can I do about the pain?

What you describe is called *central post-stroke pain*. It used to be called thalamic pain because it was believed to develop only after a stroke affecting a small part of the brain called the thalamus. Now it is realised that it can happen after any sort of stroke and usually develops, as you describe, a few months later. It is not understood why it happens in some people and not others, but it is not due to another stroke. The pain is felt as a burning or shooting sensation and can be very unpleasant. Sometimes it is triggered by movement or something touching the skin, and can occur both during the day and at night.

Treatment is difficult, but about 70% of cases can be improved at least to some extent with drugs. The earlier the treatment is started, the greater the chance of success. The drugs used most often are the tricyclic antidepressant group, amitriptyline being the first choice in most cases. These drugs are not used because the doctors think the pain is due to depression, although it is not surprising and not uncommon for depression to happen at the same time as central post-stroke pain. Amitriptyline will be started at a low dose, to try to prevent side effects, and then be gradually increased until either the pain is brought under control or the side effects become intolerable. It may be necessary to increase the dose to 100 or 150mg per day. Try to stay on the drug for at least a few weeks before giving up. The side effects, particularly drowsiness, will often improve once your body gets used to it. The other common side effect is a dry mouth, which can sometimes be helped by sips of water, sucking boiled sweets or, if necessary, artificial saliva. If amitriptyline is unsuccessful, it is worth trying one of the other tricyclic antidepressants such as maprotiline. Some doctors try anticonvulsant drugs such as carbamazepine (Tegretol), but there is little evidence to suggest that they are of much use.

A drug that has proved effective in some people is mexilitene, which was originally developed to correct irregular heart beats. It can cause your blood pressure to drop and for this reason it is usually started in hospital. You would need to be admitted for a couple of days so that they can keep an eye on you. If there are no problems then, it is perfectly safe for you to continue taking the drug at home. Gabapentin has recently been helpful for some people.

Ordinary pain-killers have very little to offer. Even the very strong pain-killers such as morphine don't seem to work and are more likely to cause additional problems.

Drug treatment is the most likely way that your pain will be helped, but if you are one of the unlucky minority who don't get any relief, it is worth experimenting with alternative treatment. Acupuncture helps some people. Transcutaneous electrical nerve stimulation (TENS) – a technique whereby tiny electrical impulses are applied by a battery-run machine attached to the skin – is worth a try. Your physiotherapy department may have a machine that you can borrow to see if it works for you. They can be bought from some chemists and surgical equipment shops for about £50. Massage is unlikely to produce lasting benefit but may give temporary relief. Learning relaxation techniques or yoga may help you cope better with the pain.

Many hospitals have specialist pain clinics; if you have had no success with your own doctor, ask to be referred to one. A few centres in the UK run in-patient pain clinics for people whose pain will not go away with the usual treatments (intractable pain), where the objective is less to kill the pain and more to help you live with the pain. Treatment is given by a multi-disciplinary team that includes physiotherapists, psychologists and physicians. If nothing else works, a referral to one of these units is justified . . . though the waiting list might be very long.

My shoulder has been very sore and stiff since the stroke. It doesn't seem to be getting better.

The shoulder joint is not very well designed. The bone of the upper arm (humerus) is held in place at the shoulder blade (scapula) by the action of the muscles around the shoulder and the fibrous bands, called ligaments, around the joint. If the muscles of the arm become paralysed, the only things holding the joint together are the ligaments, which can easily become stretched and damaged. Even just leaving the arm dangling down the side of the chair can cause injury from the weight of the arm pulling on the shoulder. More likely still to cause damage is awkward handling by the nursing staff and others who need to move you after the stroke. If just one person tries to pull you up by tugging on your arm, you can end up with a painful shoulder. Once the damage is done the symptoms are like those of a 'frozen shoulder'. It will be stiff and painful to move, and the pain can continue for up to two years. It is therefore vital that everyone who is looking after you knows about the potential problem with the shoulder joint, how to lift and handle you and the best positions in which to place your arm. This includes any friends and family who may want to help with the physical caring. The most sensitive time for the shoulder is in the first few days when the muscles are usually very floppy or flaccid. Once the 'tone' of the muscles begins to return, particularly if the muscles start becoming stiff, the risks fall significantly.

Treatment of a shoulder that has become painful is with simple pain-killers such as paracetamol or one of the anti-inflammatory drugs such as ibuprofen (Nurofen) or diclofenac (Voltarol). It used to be believed that injecting the joint with a steroid was helpful but recent research suggests that it does not work and should therefore not be used. Preventing further damage by keeping your arm well positioned is crucial. Some special straps (cuffs) are designed to keep the arm supported at the shoulder. Unfortunately, they are difficult to put on properly, can be uncomfortable to wear and probably don't work anyway. What they can do, though, is remind staff that the shoulder is at risk and should be treated with care.

I often have headaches. Is this a warning sign that I might have another stroke?

No. Headache very rarely precedes stroke, although it can happen when a stroke is actually happening. In fact, the brain itself does not have any pain sensors, so it is possible for a surgeon to operate on the brain without any anaesthetic, because the patient will not be able to feel anything! The membranes on the surface of the brain can detect painful stimuli but these membranes are rarely affected by stroke.

It is natural to attribute all symptoms to the stroke, but just as you probably used to get headaches from time to time before the stroke, so you are likely to continue to get them after the stroke. Even if you were not prone to headaches before, there is no reason to blame the stroke now.

There are lots of reasons why people get headaches, most of them having nothing to do with serious disease. Tension headaches are perhaps the commonest, which may be due to spasm of the muscles in the neck. Arthritis in the neck can also cause a similar sort of headache. Migraine can occasionally develop late in life, and if you had it before you can get it again. Sinus problems will cause headache or facial pain. Some drugs used after stroke can produce headache as a side effect. These include dipyridamole (Persantin) which is used as a treatment to prevent further stroke, some of the treatments for high blood pressure and angina such as nifedipine (Adalat), isosorbide mononitrate and glyceryl trinitrate (GTN). Often it is simply not possible to identify a cause for the pain. What many people worry about when they get a headache is that they have a brain tumour. You have probably had a recent brain scan following your stroke. If there was a tumour there, it would have been found then.

If you get a headache, take two paracetamol tablets and lie down, and it will probably go away. If it persists or keeps coming back, you should see your doctor to get the problem sorted out.

My hip and knee on my good side have started really hurting when I walk. Why is this?

What might be happening is that you are putting more strain on your good leg as a result of the weakness on the side affected by the stroke. You may be using muscles that you didn't use much before and they are objecting. Osteoarthritis of the hip and knee, which is simply due to wear and tear on the joints, is very common in older people, particularly if they have subjected their joints to heavy use in the past. If you are overweight or if you are keen on sports, particularly football, rugby, gymnastics and athletics, your joints may wear out more quickly. If you then put more pressure on the joints by limping, you may suddenly become aware that there is a problem.

Get your hip and knee examined by a doctor to establish the cause of the pain. If it is due to arthritis in the joints, the first thing to do is to consult the physiotherapist to see if anything can be done to improve the way you walk. Sometimes this will involve more exercises. Sometimes adapting your footwear can produce a remarkable relief of symptoms. You may be advised to try using a walking stick to take some of your weight. Simple pain-killers such as paracetamol can be very effective but they are usually better taken regularly rather than just occasionally – pain is easier to keep away than to get rid of when it arises. If paracetamol doesn't help, a mild anti-inflammatory drug such as ibuprofen (Nurofen) is worth trying. These can be bought over the counter (without a prescription) but should be avoided if you have, or have had, stomach ulcers. If you do buy them, ask for ibuprofen (the 'generic' name) rather than Nurofen (a trade name). It's exactly the same but cheaper.

If the arthritis is severe, it is unlikely that pain-killers on their own will be enough to keep you pain free. Then it is worth considering having the affected joint replaced. Hip replacement is very effective and the fact that you have had a stroke does not automatically bar you from an operation. Knee replacement is slightly trickier, but the artificial joints are getting better all the time and can be a great success. In the end, only you can decide whether the pain is bad enough to make you want to go through an operation. There is nothing to be lost by getting the opinion of an orthopaedic surgeon. You don't have to take their advice.

I often get painful cramps in my legs at night which wake me up. What can I do?

Night cramps happen in many people, whether or not they have had a stroke. They are more common after stroke if the muscles have developed some stiffness (spasticity). Try sleeping in a different position and change your position frequently during the night. When cramp does develop, stretch the affected muscle by bending the joint; for example, if the cramp is in your calf, pull your foot up towards the knee. This will usually produce rapid relief of the pain. If you are fortunate enough to have someone immediately available to give the muscle a massage, this is often very soothing, particularly if they use one of the relaxing aromatherapy oils. Some people find that a quinine tablet taken at bed time produces some benefit, although there is no strong scientific evidence that it does much good.

If the cause of the cramp is stiffness in the muscle, it's worth trying a muscle relaxant such as baclofen, small doses of diazepam (Valium) and tizanidine. Unfortunately, all these drugs can have side effects, so they must be taken under the direction of your doctor.

My hand gets very swollen and painful. What is this due to and what can be done?

It is quite common for the hand to swell after a stroke, and this can cause both pain and problems with regaining normal hand function. It is probably due to your hand being immobile. To keep the fluid that is normally present in your tissues circulating, you need to keep your muscles moving. If your hand is paralysed this doesn't happen, so the fluid accumulates. This will be made worse if your hand is allowed to hang down, because then the fluid has to fight gravity as well. The situation is like having painful swollen feet after a long coach or plane journey, where you have been sitting in cramped conditions for a long time.

The main treatment is to keep your hand up on a cushion in front of you. Sometimes wearing a tight glove will help to squeeze the fluid out of your hand and back into the circulation. The physiotherapist may also have a machine called a Flowtron; this is a plastic tube that fits round your arm or leg and is inflated and deflated every 10–15 minutes to squeeze the fluid out the tissues. Simple pain-killers such as paracetamol may be helpful, but ultimately the best treatment is to get your hand moving again by working hard with the physiotherapist.

A rare cause of a painful swollen hand is the 'shoulder–hand syndrome' or 'reflex sympathetic dystrophy'. We don't really understand why this develops but the main symptoms are pain on moving the shoulder, swelling in the hand and changes in the temperature of the arm, which may feel either hot or cold. The arm may look pale with dry skin. (The treatment for this is either injecting a chemical into the sympathetic nerves at the top of the arm, to stop them working, or doing a small operation to cut the nerves.)

Sensation

What can be done about the constant tingling like pins and needles that I have down the right-hand side of my face?

If the tingling developed after the stroke, it is probably due to some involvement of the part of your brain responsible for detecting sensation in your face. Unfortunately, it is unlikely that any treatment will have much effect. The drugs that help central post-stroke pain (described earlier in the section 'Pain') can be tried, but the side effects may be worse than the tingling and there is no guarantee that they will work. Using a transcutaneous electrical nerve stimulator (TENS) would be worth a go. Just as the weakness can improve after stroke, so can the sensory symptoms. We don't understand why, but sensation often recovers more slowly than movement, so don't give up hope.

I can't feel anything down my right side at all since my stroke. What can I do to speed up my recovery?

There are no treatments that have been proven to help in this situation. You may well find that, with a bit of time, the sensation does start to gradually return. In the meantime, the most important thing to do is to make sure that you don't accidentally injure yourself. Without normal pain sensation, you can easily burn yourself without knowing it or get ulcers on your feet due to poorly fitting shoes or injure your joints by getting them into positions that you wouldn't dream of if you were aware of what you were doing. So, without the feeling of pain, you have to use all your other senses to look after yourself. Always try to be aware of what your right side is doing. Watch with your eyes. Before you get in the bath, feel the temperature with your left hand. If you smoke, give up; if you can't give up, at least hold the cigarette in your left hand so you don't end up trying to inhale the smoke from your burning fingers!

My partner doesn't seem to acknowledge her left-hand side and just lets her arm dangle down, not making any effort to look after it even though the nurse keeps reminding her how important it is.

The medical term for this is *hemi-neglect*, and it usually occurs when the parietal lobe is affected by the stroke. It can be very severe, and then the problems of mood and memory described in Chapter 7 can arise. When the neglect is less severe, it may just manifest itself by the person forgetting where the arm or leg is, as you describe in your partner. She may leave her arm dangling down the side of the chair, and it is quite possible for the arm to get caught up in the spokes of her wheelchair. Her leg may keep slipping off the foot-plates of her wheelchair, ending up in awkward positions. She may repeatedly slump over to one side, unaware that she is not sitting up straight.

It is very important to identify this sort of neglect early on. Constantly reminding her that her left side exists will help her become more aware of it. If she isn't aware that she has a left

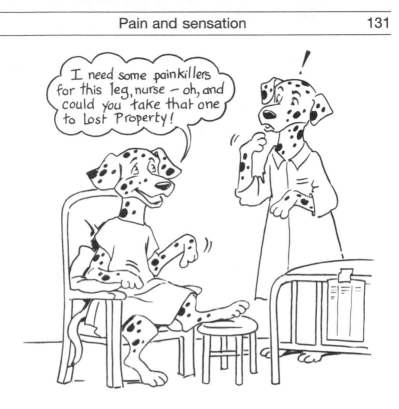

side, she won't make any effort to use it. She may even be completely unaware, unless reminded, that she has had a stroke affecting her left side and therefore will not recognise that she has to work to recover. Another problem that may arise is that her limbs can be injured, particularly at the shoulder, if they are kept in awkward positions for long periods. Or they may end up developing stiffness in certain groups of muscles that will slow up her progress in physiotherapy.

Your partner might benefit from spending some time sitting in front of a mirror, which gives her a visual reminder that she has a left side. Fitting a wide armrest onto the wheelchair to support her arm will make it less likely that it will fall to the side. The physiotherapist and occupational therapist will be working on the problem during each therapy session and it would probably be worth your attending some of the sessions to see what is being done and to get advice on what you can do to help.

9
The senses

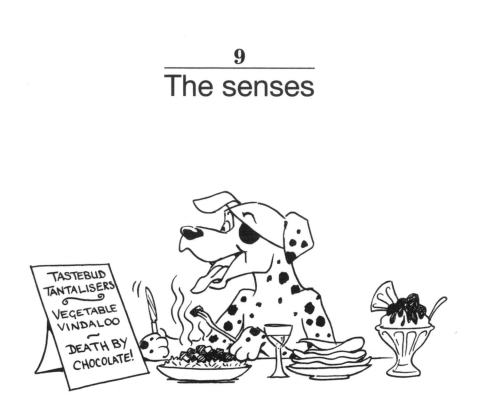

Our brain works by receiving information from our five senses – sight, sound, touch, smell and taste. Without our senses we would be totally isolated from the environment, living a life that contained nothing of value. Worse than a cabbage. This chapter describes the ways in which our senses can be affected by stroke and the ways in which problems with our senses can be overcome. We humans can be incredibly resourceful: if one sense isn't working properly, we find ways of using our remaining senses to compensate.

Vision

Why am I having difficulty seeing? Should I get my glasses changed?

Stroke can affect your vision in two main ways. If the blood clot caused a blockage of the artery to your eye, this will have damaged the retina at the back of your eye – causing partial or complete loss of vision on that side. In this case, glasses will not help, as all they can do is to correct problems with the lens and improve your ability to focus. The more common problem is for the stroke to cause damage to the nerve fibres that carry the information from the eye to the back of the brain in the occipital lobe where the information is processed. Because some of the nerve fibres from the eye cross over to the other side of the brain, all the visual information from your right side is processed in the left side of the brain, and all the information coming from the left side goes to the right half of the brain. So if your stroke involved the left half of the brain, you will lose all or some of the vision on your right side when you are looking straight ahead, and vice versa. This is called a *hemianopia*. Again, glasses will do nothing to correct this abnormality and there is no point in wasting money trying to change yours.

It is possible, of course, that the problems with your eyes have nothing to do with your stroke, and might be easily treated. So it is worth getting your optometrist or an eye specialist (ophthalmologist) to check for you.

How long will it take for my eyesight to get better?

As with the other problems following stroke, it is very difficult to make accurate predictions about the likely speed or extent of recovery. Some people do regain normal vision, while others are left with a permanent loss. If the loss of vision is complete on one side, it is likely that only about 20% of people will have fully regained their vision by one month; if there is only partial loss of vision to one side, about 75% will be back to normal in about a month.

If we look straight ahead, we will normally be aware of things going on a long way over to both our left and right sides. All that we can see like this is called the 'field of vision'. Even if your loss of vision is irreversible, with time it can become much less of a problem by your learning to scan into the damaged field of vision using your unaffected side. This means that you will have to turn your head or move your eyes a lot more than you used to and that you must always be aware that you are not going to see things so easily on one side. This is particularly important when you are in places you don't know or when you are outside. Checking carefully to right and left before crossing the road is one instance where you must concentrate to avoid risk.

I still find it difficult to read a book. Parts of the text just don't seem to be there. Is there any therapy that can help me recover my sight fully?

There are no techniques that have been proven to improve recovery from stroke-related visual problems. There are ways, though, of reducing the problems. Going back to the childhood technique of using your finger to trace each line of text can help you make sure that you read *all* the page. Using a ruler under each line can have the same effect. If you have lost your left field of vision, finding your way back to the beginning of the next line can be a problem. Use a brightly coloured marker to draw a line down the left side of the page; this will help guide your eye back to the left-hand margin and the beginning of the next line. At least to begin with, try using the large-print books available from libraries.

Special lenses have been developed that shift the images from the damaged field of vision into the normal field. These are not widely available, and can be very difficult to get used to. Until they have been tested more extensively, they should be used with caution.

The more you practise, the better you will become at dealing with the problem.

My son doesn't seem to be able to see anything to one side and isn't even aware that I sitting there. Why is this?

All the information the eyes receive from the right side of vision is processed in the left-hand side of the brain, and vice versa. So if the left side of the brain has been damaged by the stroke, the nerve fibres transmitting the visual information may have been involved, leading to right-sided blindness. The medical term for this is *homonymous hemianopia*. It is not due to a problem with the eye itself, which is only rarely affected by a stroke. There is no point therefore at this stage trying new glasses or seeing an optometrist or eye specialist. The hemianopia can recover in just the same way that, for example, people can recover strength in a paralysed limb.

If people are aware that they can't see to one side, they can compensate by turning their head or moving their eyes to the affected side. It sounds as though your son is unaware of the problem and therefore doesn't try to overcome it. This is called *visual neglect*. It is worth trying to draw his attention to his 'neglect', perhaps by always sitting on his affected side when you visit and talking to him to attract his attention. The nurses may position his bed so that most of the activity going on in the ward is happening on his blind side, again encouraging him be more aware of his 'neglect'.

Ever since the stroke, I've been seeing double. Is it likely to get any better? What can be done?

Strokes, particularly those affecting the brainstem, can cause difficulties with eye movements. Sometimes the problem is in moving both eyes in a particular direction and sometimes it is just one affected eye that doesn't move with the other one (in synchrony). It is this latter problem that most commonly results in double vision – and often resolves within a few days or weeks. During that time, covering one eye with a patch will give you relief.

Special glasses with a prism lens can sometimes be of help. The lenses bend the light reaching the weak eye, compensating for the eye's inability to bend the light itself. An optometrist or ophthalmologist will be able to advise whether these would be appropriate for you.

Taste and smell

Since my stroke, the food just doesn't taste right. Everything seems bland and I have lost my appetite as a result.

Stroke is not often recognised as causing problems with taste or smell. Although it may be the problem in your case, have you considered other possible causes? Sometimes infections such as thrush or dental caries in the mouth can affect taste. Deficiency of zinc may cause loss of taste, so if you have not been eating a balanced diet recently it might be worth taking a zinc supplement for two weeks. Some prescribed drugs cause loss of taste or abnormal tastes, so ask your doctor to check whether any of the medicines you are taking could be responsible.

Try experimenting with different flavours and smells to see if there are any that you can detect and then use those when you are preparing food. If you like spicy food, try increasing the quantities you use (so long as you don't expect anyone else to eat it!). It is important to eat a balanced diet after a stroke, both to keep you healthy now and to prevent further strokes in the future. Even if you don't feel much like eating, try to force yourself. Treat food like the medicine your doctor has prescribed – you take it even though it doesn't taste all that good.

Hearing and balance

Why have I become deaf in my right ear since the stroke?

Sudden deafness in one ear is unusual but occasionally happens after stroke. It is probably more common than doctors realise, but bedside testing of hearing is not done very frequently and, in any case, is very crude. Moreover, people are seldom sent off to the audiometry department to have formal hearing tests.

The part of the brain most likely to have been affected in your case is the brainstem, where the nerves from the inner ear enter. You should seek advice from an ear, nose and throat (ENT) specialist, if only to make sure that there is no other cause of deafness such as an infection or inner ear disease.

I feel dizzy all the time, particularly when I turn my head. Will this go away, and are there any drugs I can take to improve it in the meantime?

It is more likely that this symptom is due to inner ear problems rather than stroke. There are a number of conditions that cause *vertigo* as you describe, most of which are mild and tend to clear up within a few days. These include viral infections of the inner ear. Short-term use of drugs such as prochlorperazine (Stemetil) or betahistine (Serc) may be helpful, but you should not carry on with these drugs long term, because they can cause severe side effects. Sometimes strokes affecting the cerebellum or brainstem can produce an abnormal sensation of movement, but this rarely persists for long.

10
Living with disability

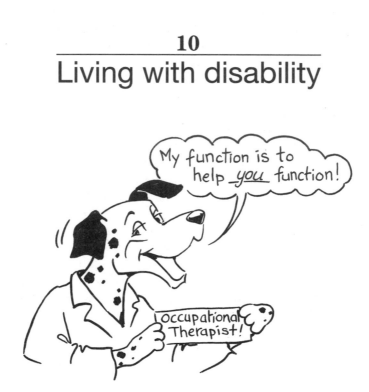

Occupational therapists (OTs) are there to help you to make the best possible use of the function that you are left with after the stroke by giving you exercises and providing you with special equipment. The multiple and almost limitless roles of the occupational therapist mean that there are rarely enough of them to be able to do everything that is desirable, but knowing how they can help you will enable you to know what to ask for.

The first stage is to do a detailed assessment of what your problems are. This will not just be in terms of what movement you have in your hands, arms and legs but also whether you have any difficulties with sensation and perception. You may, for example, not be fully aware of what your body can or cannot do. The occupational therapist will assess your memory and ability to learn new tasks, sometimes working with the psychologist. The assessments should start within the first few days of your stroke and will be done in conjunction with all the other members of the stroke team.

Early on, the occupational therapist will give advice on and provide equipment that will make your life easier. This may include sorting out the chair you are sitting on so that it gives you the most appropriate degree of support and the best cushion for you to sit on comfortably without getting pressure sores. If you have a paralysed hand, you may benefit from cutlery that can be used with one hand and a non-slip plate mat so that the plate doesn't slide off the table when you eat. You may need a 'plate guard' so that the food stays on the plate while you cut it or try to pick it up with a fork.

The occupational therapist will often concentrate on your hand and arm function. Movement in the hand is commonly one of the last things to come back after a stroke, and it is very important not to let it get stiff or swollen when it is paralysed. You may be given exercises to do. Sometimes you may need to wear a splint on your hand to prevent your fingers from curling up, or have a special tight glove to stop the swelling.

As movement returns, the occupational therapist will be working with you to improve your function in the 'activities of daily living' (ADL). So they may take you to the kitchen to practise making simple meals or that essential cup of tea. If necessary, they will teach you how to wash and dress yourself – which can be extraordinarily difficult with a paralysed arm or clumsy fingers. Doing up buttons with one hand may be made easier by putting Velcro fastenings on your clothes. If you can't get into the bath or shower easily, you may need an aid or equipment to help you wash in front of a basin; for example, a flannel on the end of a flexible stick may enable you to wash your back. If you have a weak leg, getting up from a low toilet seat may not be feasible; the occupational therapist can provide a raised toilet seat. For nearly every problem there is some gadget or clever technique that may make an impossible task merely difficult.

As the time approaches for you to go home the occupational therapist will be helping you prepare for this. You may need a visit home before you are discharged from hospital, to assess the environment and decide on changes needed to make your life easier. The occupational therapist's job doesn't stop when you get home. Even though living independently may have been made possible by the provision of various aids and appliances, you will probably discover other problems when you are back home. In the longer term the plan must be to get you functioning as near normally as possible. This means stopping using your aids as soon as they are no longer essential.

Occupational therapy is not just about getting you to perform the basic activities of daily living. It is also about getting you to regain as many as possible of the higher level skills that you had before, such as cooking, drawing or playing the guitar again. Getting you back to work, for example, might mean taking you out to sweep up leaves if you were a street sweeper, or redeveloping keyboard skills if you were an office worker, and so on.

Major illnesses often present the individuals affected, and their families and friends, with particular challenges, and some adjustments may be needed in order to return to successful community living. The nature and extent of the changes that may be necessary are likely to depend on the level and degree of impairment resulting from your stroke and whether these are long term or permanent. Not everyone who has a stroke will need counselling, but you might well find it useful to see a counsellor for a limited period in order to explore issues concerning the nature and meaning of your illness and its longer term effects.

Occupational therapy

How soon after my stroke should I see the occupational therapist?

The occupational therapist will need to get involved as soon as you begin your rehabilitation. If you are quite ill at the beginning and are spending much of your day in bed, most of the treatment will be given by the doctors, nurses and physiotherapists, and the occupational therapist will not have a big role. Once you are sitting out of bed and beginning to try doing things for yourself, though, the occupational therapist will be needed to give advice on the most appropriate ways of helping you improve.

It seems to me that the occupational therapist and the physiotherapist are working against each other. The physiotherapist is trying to get me moving properly and the occupational therapist is teaching me ways around my difficulties in moving. Shouldn't I wait until I see what I'll never be able to do and then see the OT?

The occupational therapist and physiotherapist work together as a team and, while of course the aim is to get you back completely to normal, this may not be possible. In any case, in the meantime you should be working to be as independent as possible. Nothing the occupational therapist does will stop you from recovering, and any equipment provided can (and should) be removed when you no longer need it. You will probably need to learn new skills to get around any difficulties that remain, and the earlier you begin to learn these the better. It would be much harder to learn them later, particularly when you are out of hospital without easy access to intensive therapy.

The OT has mentioned a home visit. What is this for?

Before you are discharged from hospital, it is often useful for you to have a visit home with the occupational therapist. This will enable you to get some idea of how you will manage when you are at home again. It will also provide some ideas about possible problem areas. The occupational therapist will be able to advise on any special equipment that might help you – in the kitchen, the bathroom or any other living area. The therapist will also be able to check safety aspects such as loose carpets, the need for extra stair rails and so forth. Sometimes the occupational therapist will first visit your home without you, just to look around and get an idea of the skills you must have before being discharged from hospital. Closer to the time of your discharge a further visit will often be done with you to check exactly where the difficulties are. If you are going to need some help from a carer when you are home, it is helpful if your carer can be there for the visit so that they can be shown what is planned and what their role is going to be.

Aids and equipment at home

How much special equipment for disabled people is available on the NHS, and how much will I have to pay for?

A certain amount of equipment for people with impairments is available free of charge either from the NHS or from occupational therapy services provided by local authority social services departments. Such equipment is usually provided on an open-ended loan basis: once it is no longer needed, it is returned to the NHS or to social services. Items included in this type of provision are certain types of seating, aids for bathing or using the toilet, and various types of kitchen equipment such as saucepan holders or grips. Blocks to raise the height of chairs or beds can also be provided, as can stair lifts in certain circumstances (and for certain types of stairs). Sloping ramps for wheelchair access to a property or rails and handles to help with steps and doorways may also be included.

Other items that are more expensive, or that would require adaptations to the property, are likely to involve your being assessed financially (means-tested) to see if you are able to contribute to their cost. For example, you may well be expected to contribute to the cost of adapting ground floor accommodation, a shower suitable for a disabled person or a lift. In some cases, you might be assessed as being able to afford the full cost of these and would therefore be expected to pay for them yourself. Adaptations to property may be made through the local authority housing department if your accommodation is council owned. Some of the cost of such adaptations is likely to be borne by the housing department, and in any case the agreement of the housing department (as landlord) will be needed before any alteration or adaptation can be made. On the other hand, the housing department might have other accommodation available that has already been adapted for use by a disabled person and you would be offered the chance to move to such property.

How can I find out about what equipment there is?

It is part of the specialised roles of occupational therapists and physiotherapists to provide advice and guidance about aids and equipment. Whilst physiotherapists are concerned primarily with mobility and assistance with movement, occupational therapists are more involved in assistance with various aspects of daily living and helping people to function as well as possible where they live and work. Many hospital occupational and physio-therapy departments have a wide range of equipment that people can try out before they buy or hire it. They may also have catalogues of companies that specialise in such provision.

Some bigger towns have shops or showrooms displaying the equipment for you try out on the premises. The Disabled Living Centres Council (address in Appendix 1) can advise you about a Centre near you, where you can see and try out equipment. Some of the more sophisticated pieces of equipment that are not available through the social services or the health service will need to be bought privately either from the specialist shops or through the catalogues. Even if the equipment is not available free, the occupational therapist will be able to advise you on which items are worth investing in and where you can obtain them.

I'm supposed to be getting a wheelchair but it will be several weeks before it arrives. What do I do in the meantime?

If you are still in hospital, they should be able to lend you one. If you are at home, the local branch of the Red Cross will usually able to rent you one for a small fee.

I'm going to need a wheelchair but the ones the wheelchair service provide don't meet my needs. I've seen some people in chairs that are much better than the one I've been offered. How can I get one?

If you can't persuade your wheelchair service to fund a more expensive chair, you will have to pay for it yourself. They might part-fund it, with you making up the difference. Some charities will help if you have special needs; you can also try asking in your local reference library for the *Guide to Grants for Individuals in Need.*

Emotional factors

My walking is so unsteady, I feel as though everyone is staring at me when I go out. They must think I'm drunk. Because I feel embarrassed about this I stay at home. Do you have any advice?

People do stare at anyone who is a bit unusual, and unfortunately there is not much one can do to stop them. You need to develop a very thick skin. Be proud of the fact that, despite your stroke, you have managed to get back to the point where you are able to get out and look after yourself. Don't punish yourself for the ignorance of others. What does it matter if they stare? It's their problem, not yours.

I think that some counselling would help me to come to terms with the stroke. How can I go about getting this?

Some stroke or hospital rehabilitation units have direct contact with local counselling services. Others are likely to suggest and use social workers and occupational therapists or nurses who have had training for short-term counselling. An increasing number of primary care groups and health centres now have counsellors attached to them, so if you feel that it would be

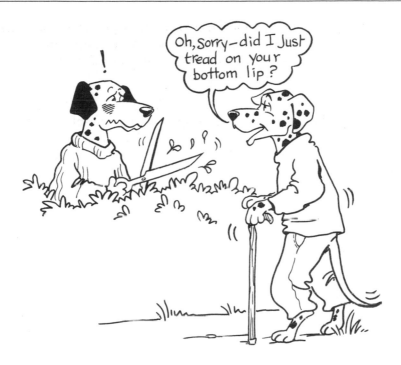

useful to see somebody once you are back home, discuss this with your GP. This would also be the case if you wished to have ongoing sessions with a counsellor or social worker over a longer period of time once you are home.

11

Why have I had a stroke and what can I do to prevent another one?

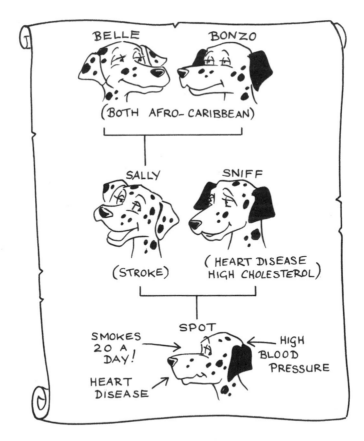

Many of the factors that make you more likely to have stroke are known, but it is still not unusual for a stroke to occur with no obvious cause. Some of these *risk factors*, such as a strong family history of stroke, are things that cannot be changed. However, high blood pressure (hypertension), diabetes (diabetes mellitus), smoking, excessive alcohol consumption, high cholesterol and obesity (being very overweight), heart disease and abnormalities of the clotting system in the blood can all be controlled to some extent so as to minimise the chance of someone having a stroke.

Risk factors for stroke

If your blood relatives have had a stroke, there is a slightly increased risk of stroke for you. This may in part be due to things such as high cholesterol being inherited but there are probably also additional genetic factors that are not yet understood. Social class seems to affect the risk of stroke (and many other illnesses): for example, people in social class 1 (professionals, such as lawyers and doctors) have a much lower frequency of stroke than those in social class 5 (unskilled workers). Ethnic group is also an important factor: people of African-Caribbean descent are at greater risk of stroke than 'white' people; in the Far East, haemorrhage (bleeding) into the brain is much more common than it is in Europe and North America. Abnormalities in the blood vessels supplying the brain (such as aneurysms or arterio-venous malformations) are things that people are born with, live with for years without any problems and then discover them only when, for some reason, they burst, allowing blood to leak into the brain – resulting in a stroke.

Are strokes hereditary?

There is a slightly increased chance of having a stroke if members of your immediate family have had strokes. This is particularly true if your relatives were young when they had their strokes.

Some of the reasons why strokes run in families are understood and relate to high cholesterol and high blood pressure being in part inherited problems. We also tend to take on certain behavioural characteristics from our families. For example, eating patterns are learnt from our parents, and high alcohol consumption and smoking may be copied from one generation to the next. Social class depends to a large extent on our parents, although obviously it can be changed.

If you have a family history of stroke, it is worth discussing this with your doctor to see if there is anything you should do to modify your lifestyle to minimise your risk. Nevertheless, even if all your close relatives had strokes, the chance of your having one is not all that great. It should not be regarded as the Sword of Damocles hanging over you, over which you have no control.

It was only recently that I was found to have high blood pressure. Why have I had a stroke so soon?

The risk of stroke, particularly haemorrhage, is highest early after you develop high blood pressure. When there is increased pressure inside the arteries, the blood vessel affected gradually responds by thickening the walls to strengthen it. This process will take months, during which time the pressure is high, and the wall is thin and can easily burst. So it is not unusual for the stroke to happen soon after the diagnosis of high blood pressure has been made. This is why it is important to have your blood pressure checked regularly, at least every year, and to take your doctor's advice about how to get the pressure down. If your blood pressure is treated effectively and is kept within normal limits, your risk of stroke is no greater than that of someone who has normal blood pressure. However, don't think that you are safe if you have survived with untreated high blood pressure for a few years. Eventually your heart will become seriously damaged and the lining of your arteries will be at much greater risk of 'furring up' with fatty deposits than those in people without high pressure. The risk, then, is that the blood flow to the brain will be blocked off and cause an infarct (damage to the brain).

Even though high blood pressure rarely causes any symptoms,

it is a dangerous condition if left untreated. Most people can be treated effectively, either with simple changes to lifestyle – losing a bit of weight, reducing salt intake or taking a bit more exercise – or by taking a drug, most of which are safe and cause few if any side effects. Even if you have already had a stroke, it is not too late to start treatment for high blood pressure. It is probably the single most important thing to do to reduce your risk of having another stroke.

What is a 'normal' blood pressure?

Humans evolved from lifestyles very different from those that most of us have today. Until very recently (in evolutionary terms) we lived in rural environments, hunting and growing our own food and probably exercising much more than the average person does now. There are not many societies that still live in this way, but evidence from those that do shows that their blood pressures are usually much lower than the 'normal' levels that we accept in developed countries. It is likely that the vast majority of people today have much higher blood pressures than we were 'designed' for. Increasingly, doctors are beginning to accept that people should try to keep their blood pressure as low as they can manage without getting symptoms of low blood pressure (dizziness, falls, fainting). You should be aiming for a blood pressure of less than 140mmHg systolic (the peak pressure reached in the arteries) and 85mmHg diastolic (the lowest pressure) regardless of your age.

To check your blood pressure, it must be measured in the correct way:

- The cuff used should be the correct size for your arm.

- The measurement should be taken while you are sitting and relaxed.

If hypertension is suspected, there should be three separate readings, all above the normal range. One high reading, particularly if it is taken while you are feeling anxious after rushing to the clinic, does not mean you have hypertension.

If your blood pressure rises and falls a lot over the course of the day and it is difficult to know what the latest reading represents, there is a machine that can be used to record your pressure automatically every 15 or 30 minutes for 24 hours. It is being used increasingly to assist in the diagnosis and management of hypertension. (Note that *hyper*tension is high blood pressure; *hypo*tension is low blood pressure.)

Is there anything – apart from taking drugs – that I can do to keep my blood pressure down?

The following are worth trying, and will bring down your blood pressure a bit.

- Lose weight if you are overweight.
- Cut down on your salt intake by not adding any extra to food once it has come to the table.
- Take more exercise.

It is reasonable to give these measures three months to work, but if after this time your pressure remains high, the drugs that are used to treat it are usually free of side effects, easy to take and effective. I [AR] strongly recommend that you take your doctor's advice and agree to use them.

Various homoeopathic and herbal remedies are available for the treatment of hypertension. As far as I am aware, none has been subjected to the sort of rigorous scientific evaluation that conventional drugs have to undergo to show that they work and are safe. If you do decide to try them, let your doctor know what you are doing; if they don't work, switch to an alternative – preferably a conventional one!

Is there any point stopping smoking now that I've already had the stroke?

Yes. The risk of your having another stroke will be reduced if you stop smoking. If you had advanced lung cancer as a result of smoking, there would be little point in giving up, but with stroke and heart attacks it is never too late. The beneficial effects start from the first day you stop. Although giving up completely is by far the best thing you can do, if you really cannot do without cigarettes, at least cut down the number you smoke.

I've tried giving up smoking before unsuccessfully. Can you help?

The first and most important stage in giving up smoking is making the decision that you really want to stop. If you are half-hearted about it or are only doing it to please someone else, you are not very likely to succeed. There are lots of good reasons why it is sensible to give up, including:

- Your risk of having another stroke – which could be very severe – will be reduced.

- The chance of your having a heart attack will be less.

- Lung disease, including cancer and emphysema, stomach cancer and ulcers, cancer of the bladder, gangrene of the feet, cancer of the throat and tongue as well as many others are all undoubtedly linked to smoking.

And then of course there is the cost! If you smoke a pack of cigarettes a day, giving up now will save you over £1600 that you can spend this time next year. Perhaps a holiday in the Caribbean to celebrate your new lease of life?

If you really have decided to give up, we suggest:

- Set a date (perhaps in two weeks) when you are going to give up.

- Keep a smoking diary to see which are your 'most important' cigarettes of the day.

- The day you stop, go and sit somewhere quiet and smoke your last cigarette. Make sure you really enjoy it.

- Then get rid of all the cigarettes, matches and lighters from the house. (If there is even one cigarette left, the temptation to have it at a moment of stress will be too great.) If you do weaken, you will have enough time to change your mind while you make your way to the tobacconist.

- The most difficult times will be when you traditionally used to light up – after a meal, with your morning coffee and so on. Try to change your routine at these times. Even a little change such as having your coffee in the kitchen instead of the living room may be enough.

- Use your smoking diary to help you plan changes to your routines.

- When you fancy a cigarette, go and do something else. In a few seconds the feeling will pass if you stop thinking about it.

- Don't allow anyone else in your house to smoke in front of you. Visitors can wait till they leave, or go outside.

- Try to persuade family members to give up in solidarity with you. Then when one of you weakens, the other can pretend to be 'holier than thou'.

- Ask one person, who understands the difficulties of giving up, to help support you.

- For at least a few weeks avoid visiting places, such as the pub, where smoking is part of the culture.

- For the rest of your life there will be times when you fancy a cigarette. Just remember how much effort it was giving up the first time! The feeling will pass.

- If the withdrawal symptoms are too much to bear, you might find that nicotine replacement therapy (NRT) can help. This comes in six different forms: a skin patch, chewing gum, a lozenge to suck, inhaler, nasal spray and a tablet that you place under your tongue. Under no circumstances should you carry on smoking and use the nicotine replacement. Your GP or practice nurse will probably be able to give you advice, and it may be possible to get a prescription for the NRT on the NHS.

- The most effective way of using nicotine replacement treatment is to combine it with some counselling or support from your doctor or a counsellor.

The NHS Smoking Helpline and the charity Quit offer information and advice about giving up smoking (contact numbers in Appendix 1).

There are a lot advertisements promoting easy ways to give up smoking, most of which require you to part with large amounts of money. There is little scientific evidence that meditation, acupuncture or any other special techniques are of much use. Unfortunately, the area has attracted a lot of people who are keen to earn some easy money from vulnerable smokers. Be careful. If you want to try something, give it limited time. If it isn't working, stop.

I have been under a lot of pressure at work. Would I have had the stroke if I hadn't been so stressed?

Stroke is usually the result of progressive damage to the arteries of the brain over the years. We don't know what effect stress has on the arteries, although it is generally believed that it does increase the risk of stroke and heart attack. Whether this is the direct result of the stress or reflects something else about the sort of people who end up getting stressed is not clear. A sudden shock can cause a surge in blood pressure, which can occasionally result in blood leaking out of the artery and producing a haemorrhage. This might have been the cause of a stroke in a lady who developed her symptoms immediately on being told that she had breast cancer. Unfortunately, there isn't much that can be done to avoid this sort of stress.

Chronic stress at work happens mainly to people who are put in positions that they are not equipped to deal with. Being in a busy, demanding job with lots of responsibility probably will not increase the risk of stroke if you are coping with it and enjoying the demands made of you. However, if you find that stress levels at work or at home are making you feel ill, get some advice about how the situation can be improved. Your manager at work, your spouse or partner, your GP, a counsellor or a good friend might all be good people to talk to.

There are several techniques that some people find useful to reduce stress levels. Meditation and yoga are well known. Finding a hobby that you enjoy and that demands a relaxed mind such as fishing or golf or even just going home and stroking your pet rabbit or cat have been shown to be helpful in reducing stress.

I have a very responsible job, supervising a lot of staff and in charge of a big budget. Before the stroke I was working long hours. My wife thinks it is time to retire, as she is worried that if I go back to work I'll end up with another stroke. What should I do?

If you were enjoying your job and were good at it, you should probably try to get back to work. But if you were finding it a strain and were in fact looking for a reason for a change in lifestyle, here it is.

If you plan to get back to work, see if it is possible to start part-time. Nearly every job has bits that you could do without. Sit down and discuss with your manager how you can make your job more satisfying. There may well be things that you used to do that someone else can do as well or better. Try to identify why your job required such long hours. Were you really using the time productively, or were you staying late at the office because you were being inefficient in some parts of your job? Or were you staying late because you felt it was expected of you, to prove your dedication to the job?

You will probably find it more difficult to get back into the routines than you anticipate, and certainly you will find yourself becoming more tired than you used to. There may also be some parts of your job that you find more difficult. Your memory may need some retraining. You may find that dealing with multiple problems all at once is much more difficult. Be prepared for some difficulties and then you won't be disappointed.

If you decide to retire when you would really rather be at work, it may well end up being more stressful, not only for you but also for your wife. There is something to be said for marriage vows to be 'in sickness and in health, but never for lunch'! On the other hand, retirement for many people is the best time of their lives. But it won't be if all you plan to do is to spend 30 years sitting in an armchair watching soap operas!

Could my stroke have been prevented if the doctor had realised I'd had a TIA?

TIAs, or transient ischaemic attacks, are strokes that recover completely within 24 hours. In fact the majority last only a few minutes. The causes are exactly the same as for strokes that don't improve within 24 hours, and they need to be investigated and treated in the same way. The highest risk of going on to develop a stroke is within the first few days, so don't delay in seeking medical help. If your TIA had been recognised and preventive treatment given, it is possible that your present stroke might not have happened. Even with the best treatment, however, only about a third of strokes are prevented, so there is certainly no guarantee that you would now be well.

What tests should I have done if I have a TIA?

The most important thing is to have a history taken of what happened by someone experienced in assessing people with TIA. There are lots of symptoms that are initially thought by the general public or GPs to be TIA but are not.

If the specialist thinks a TIA is likely, it may be that he or she will want to get a brain scan done, although not always. Many people will need an ultrasound examination of the blood flow through the carotid arteries (the main blood vessels taking blood to the brain). You will need to have some blood taken to check that your blood count and blood chemistry are normal and you should have your cholesterol checked. A tracing of your heart (electrocardiogram) and perhaps an echocardiogram will also be done.

What should I do if I have one TIA after another?

Our advice is that if you have two or more TIAs within a few days you should be investigated urgently. That may require you to spend a day or two in hospital. Don't ignore them. By definition they will get better on their own but the next one could be a stroke and not a TIA!

My husband and I were fighting so much before the stroke that I feel guilty. Could I have caused the stroke?

A sudden rise in blood pressure can very occasionally trigger a stroke. In most instances, though, it is likely that if the stroke had not happened after your argument it would have happened the next day or the day after, without a fight. There is no point and probably no reason to feel guilty.

Nevertheless, it would probably be a good idea to use this as an opportunity to try to sort out your relationship, as you both need to be as supportive of each other as possible over the coming months. If you find that it is difficult to talk openly to each other, think about getting some help from a third party. Relate (contact details in Appendix 1) is a charity devoted to helping people with relationship problems, or your GP might be able to point you in the right direction.

Years ago I was told I had a heart murmur. Was my stroke due to this, and should something have been done then?

Sometimes heart murmurs signify important heart disease that needs attention, but many people have heart murmurs that are of no significance and need no treatment. Sorting out what sort of murmur you have is the job of your doctor, who may want to seek the opinion of a heart specialist (cardiologist) or have some tests done. A murmur is the sound that can be heard, through a stethoscope, that the blood makes when the flow through the heart is turbulent rather than smooth. This can occur if one of the heart valves fails to open or close efficiently or sometimes if there is abnormal flow of blood between the chambers of the heart.

Some murmurs do indicate heart disease that can cause stroke. They include the murmurs of *mitral stenosis* or *aortic stenosis* (narrowing of the valves on the left side of the heart) and *ventricular septal defect* (a hole in the muscle separating the two main chambers of the heart). All of these are uncommon, but it is likely that they would have been identified at the time of your stroke and you would have been told about them. Ask your doctor whether you still have a murmur and what it is due to. If there is any uncertainty, it would be worth asking the opinion of a cardiologist.

My brother-in-law, who is from Jamaica, was told that stroke is more common in people from the Caribbean. Why is this?

Recent evidence has shown that the risk of a stroke is about twice as high for an African-Caribbean person living in London as for a 'white' person. We don't know exactly why this is so. It may be partly due to high blood pressure and diabetes being more prevalent in African-Caribbean people in the UK. Their blood pressure may not be treated as effectively either, as it often does not respond well to some of the commonly used drugs. There may also be some other genetic or environmental factors that have yet to be identified, and research is underway to try to identify these.

My son was only admitted for an investigation on his heart, following a recent heart attack, and he had a stroke during the test. What went wrong?

There is a close link between heart disease and stroke. Both are usually due to 'furring up' of the blood vessels, so it is not surprising that the two often coexist. Unfortunately, there is a small risk of stroke associated with investigations that involve the insertion of a catheter (a narrow tube) into the heart. The catheter can dislodge a blood clot sitting inside one of the chambers of the heart, which then gets carried to the brain and causes a stroke. The chance of this happening is less than one in a hundred, and for most people will be more than offset by the possible benefits of sorting out their heart problem.

The risks of any procedure would have been explained to your son before he signed his consent for it to be carried out. The problem is that there is no way of knowing in advance who is going to suffer the disadvantages. We all go through life playing the equivalent of the lottery with our health. There are ways of increasing of the odds of winning, such as avoiding things that are known to be harmful (e.g. smoking), but even if we lead a perfect life we cannot avoid all risk.

I've got an irregular heart rhythm. Shouldn't this have been treated before to prevent me having a stroke?

The normal heart rhythm is regular, speeding up and slowing down a little with your breathing and getting faster when you exercise or get excited. There are several reasons why your heart might start beating irregularly. It is very common for there to be occasional extra beats called *extrasystoles*. They are completely safe, happen in everyone sometimes, and usually go unnoticed except perhaps for a slight *palpitation* (uncomfortable awareness of the heart beat). They happen more often in people who use a lot of stimulants such as tea or coffee. There is no link with stroke, and can be safely ignored.

If your heart starts beating irregularly all the time, it is possible that it has gone into *atrial fibrillation* (caused by the part of the heart that acts as a pacemaker not working properly). In the general population, about 5% of people are 'in atrial fibrillation'. Of those who have a stroke, nearly a quarter are in atrial fibrillation. The heart can carry on pumping without much loss of efficiency in atrial fibrillation but there is a small increased risk of stroke. This risk can be reduced by either taking one aspirin tablet every day or, better still, taking an anticoagulant such as warfarin. There are some people for whom warfarin is not appropriate and the best treatment for you will need to be discussed with your doctor. If you were in atrial fibrillation before the stroke and it was known about and left untreated, you are right in thinking that your treatment was not ideal. There would have been no guarantee that the aspirin or warfarin would have prevented your stroke but the chances of it happening would have been much less.

Everyone should learn how to feel their own pulse. The easiest place to find it is at the wrist. Place your index finger gently on the underside of your wrist at the thumb side and you should be able to feel the radial artery pulsating. Its position can vary a little between individuals, so just move your finger around a bit if at first you can't feel anything. The other places it is easy to feel the pulse are in the neck and the groin. Only ever feel one side of your neck at a time, as it is possible to stop your heart by rubbing both carotid arteries at once! The pulse can be felt just to one side of your windpipe and Adam's apple. If, having felt your pulse, you think it is beating irregularly, don't panic! Arrange to see your doctor some time in the next few weeks. Unless there is a good reason not to, you should take one aspirin (300mg) tablet a day until your appointment.

I've been told that my stroke might be something to do with my snoring. How can this be?

Snoring is sometimes a sign of a condition called *sleep apnoea*. If you have this, your normal breathing pattern during sleep is disturbed, and there are periods of up to about half a minute when your breathing stops. This disrupts your sleep because every time you go into a deep sleep your brain has to wake you up to get you to start breathing again. As a result, you wake in the morning feeling tired and you cat nap during the day. The condition tends to occur in people who are very overweight (obese), but this is not always the case. There is some evidence, although more research is needed, to suggest that sleep apnoea makes a person more likely to have stroke and heart disease.

The only way for the condition to be diagnosed accurately is to have a sleep study done in one of the few sleep centres in the UK. Here they will attach various monitors to you that record your brain waves, breathing, eye movements and heart rate, and observe you overnight while you sleep. If the condition is confirmed, the treatment is for you to sleep using oxygen through a facemask. The oxygen supply is attached to a machine that senses when your breathing has stopped and fills your lungs with air so that the oxygen level in your blood doesn't fall. This is called *non-invasive positive-pressure ventilation* (NIPPV). Going to sleep with the mask on takes some getting used to, but it can transform your life, giving you much more energy during the day. If you have sleep apnoea, treating it could also prevent another stroke. A lot more research is needed in this area, but it will probably become a very important treatment in the future.

I've had diabetes for years. Could this be why I've had a stroke?

Diabetes is one of the major risk factors for stroke. It causes the build-up of fatty deposits in the arteries, particularly the smaller arteries in the brain, and increases the chances of these blood vessels becoming blocked and causing a stroke. This is most likely if you have had diabetes for many years, especially if your blood sugar has not been tightly controlled. It can occur with both types of diabetes – that in younger people who have to use insulin (Type 1) and the type that starts in older people, who don't have to use insulin (maturity onset, non-insulin-dependent diabetes; Type 2). The long-held belief that good control of diabetes results in fewer complications such as stroke has recently been confirmed in research studies.

I have been taking the oral contraceptive – 'the Pill'. Was having a stroke due to this?

Stroke in women of child-bearing age is very uncommon. In a few of these 'the Pill' may have contributed to the cause. The risk of stroke in women taking the low-dose oestrogen oral contraceptive is about twice that of women not using it. There is no evidence of any increased risk using the progesterone-only pill. Although doubling the risk may seem very high, the number of young women having a stroke is so low that the actual increase in the number of strokes is very small indeed. The risk of having a stroke or heart attack because you use an oral contraceptive is increased if you have high blood pressure, are over 35 years of age and smoke. Therefore, many family planning clinics now recommend that women stop taking the combined pill at 35 if they have any additional risk factors for stroke or heart disease. Certainly now that you have had a stroke, we would advise you not to go back on the pill but to discuss with your doctor other means of contraception.

I was using hormone replacement therapy (HRT). Could this have caused the stroke?

Recent evidence suggests that women taking HRT have a slightly higher risk of developing stroke and heart attacks. There are lots of reasons to take HRT but preventing stroke is not one of them. Few studies so far have looked at the overall risks and benefits of taking long-term HRT. It undoubtedly prevents the development of osteoporosis (fragile bones) and resultant fractures in later life. It is highly effective at helping prevent symptoms such as hot flushes that women often suffer around the time of the menopause, but there is an increased risk of not just stroke and heart disease but also breast cancer and cancer of the womb. Most doctors now advise women to use HRT for only a few years after the menopause and if they have had a stroke while on HRT to stop taking it.

I'm only 28 and have had a stroke. Are there any causes that the doctors should look for that might explain what has happened?

All the causes of stroke in older people can also happen in young people. There is also, however, a long list of rare conditions that very occasionally can cause stroke in young people. Because the disease is unusual in someone of your age, you should be sent (referred) to a specialist in neurology or stroke medicine for further assessment. The sorts of conditions that can result in stroke fall into one of four kinds:

- abnormalities of the blood vessels to the brain,

- problems in the blood that make it more likely that the arteries will become blocked with clot,

- problems related to blood pressure,

- diseases of the heart.

PROBLEMS WITH THE ARTERIES

Arterial problems are mainly related to disease of the wall of the vessel. If there is weakness of the collagen – which is the protein that gives the wall its strength – an aneurysm can form. Alternatively, the blood can get between the layers of collagen to cause what is called a *dissection* of the artery. This can either result in the blood escaping from the artery into the brain or else cause a blood clot to form in the artery. Dissection of the artery can also result from trauma: for example, a whiplash injury can sometimes result not only in a painful neck but also in a dissection of the carotid or vertebral arteries. Dissection can occur for no very clear reason or from very minor injury. For example, someone recently sustained a dissection simply from turning his head rapidly – this is very rare! Someone else developed a dissection from holding a mobile phone between his shoulder and ear for an hour.

Arterio-venous malformations are problems with the arteries that you are born with. Instead of being in an orderly arrangement, there is a mass of tangled vessels. These blood vessels are fragile and can burst for no apparent reason, causing a cerebral haemorrhage.

In some diseases the arteries become inflamed and, as a result, can close up. These are grouped under the name *vasculitis*. Many diseases can cause vasculitis, including some infections such as syphilis and meningitis. Rheumatoid arthritis and systemic lupus crythcmatosus (SLE) are two of the more common auto-immune diseases that can cause vasculitis. Cocaine has also caused vasculitis, leading to stroke.

PROBLEMS WITH THE BLOOD

The blood problems are mainly related to abnormalities of the clotting mechanism. People with sickle cell disease are at high risk of their blood forming clots in the small arteries of the brain. Severe anaemia can cause stroke. If the platelets are abnormal in function or number, there may be bleeding into the brain or clots may form in the arteries. For reasons that are not understood, the body can start fighting itself using its immune system. It produces antibodies against some of its own tissues, which can cause clots to form both in the veins of the legs and in the arteries of the brain. The most common form of this abnormality is something called *antiphospholipid* or *Hughes' syndrome*. The clotting mechanism can also become abnormal during or immediately after pregnancy, leading to a slightly increased chance of stroke.

PROBLEMS WITH THE BLOOD PRESSURE

A problem with uncontrolled blood pressure can occur at any age. One of the causes of stroke that is being seen more and more often is abuse of stimulant-like drugs such as ecstasy or amphetamines, which can cause a huge surge in blood pressure and cerebral haemorrhage.

DISEASES OF THE HEART

Arteries may become blocked with debris that has broken off from infected heart valves in the disease called *infective endocarditis*. This is most likely to occur when the heart valves are already abnormal, either from birth or caused by an infection. People who inject drugs into their veins or arteries are particularly at risk of developing infected heart valves.

Sometimes, if there is a hole between the left and right sides of the heart (e.g. patent foramen ovale), a blood clot that forms in the veins of the legs can cross over into the left side of the heart and travel up to the brain, producing a stroke.

Drugs to prevent stroke

Which are the best drugs to take to keep my blood pressure down?

The choice of drugs available for the treatment of high blood pressure is very large. The drug that is best suited to you will be one that is effective, has no side effects and, preferably, needs to be taken only once a day. Unfortunately, it is not always possible to choose the right drug first time and often there has to be a period of trial and error while different drugs are tried and doses adjusted. Sometimes it is necessary to take two or more drugs to achieve adequate control. It is likely that a drug from one of the following groups will be appropriate for you.

- Thiazide diuretics (water tablets) – e.g. bendrofluazide. Many doctors will start treatment with one of these. They work by making the body get rid of sodium through the urine. Only very small doses are needed to achieve a fall in blood pressure and, although they are water tablets, you are unlikely to be aware that you are having to go to the toilet to pass more urine. They are slow to work and you should take them for three months before deciding to switch to something else. They should be taken with care if you are susceptible to gout or if you have diabetes.

- Angiotensin-converting enzyme inhibitors (ACE inhibitors) – e.g. perindopril, ramipril, captopril, enalapril, lisinopril. These work on an enzyme system that regulates the production of a hormone responsible for the amount of sodium present in your body. They are often used in combination with a water tablet (diuretic) and in a couple of recent trials have been shown to be very effective at reducing the risk of further strokes. One of the more common side effects is a dry cough, which can sometimes be avoided by switching to one of the newer, more specific, drugs such as losartan or valsartan.

- Calcium antagonists – e.g. nifedipine, amlodipine. They act by dilating peripheral (small) blood vessels. They can cause headache and swelling of your ankles but are generally very effective and safe.

- Beta-blockers – e.g. atenolol, propranolol, sotalol, metoprolol. These are widely used, and work by slowing the heart and dilating some of the arteries, especially those to muscle. Avoid using them if you have problems with the circulation to your hands or feet or if you have asthma.

- Alpha-blockers – e.g. doxazosin. These can be highly effective, especially for people from Africa and the Caribbean whose blood pressure often does not respond to beta-blockers or the ACE inhibitors.

Why is aspirin important, and how does it work?

There are two common uses for aspirin. One is as a pain-killer and anti-inflammatory, and so is useful, for example, in arthritis or headache. This was known generations ago by some of the native Indian tribes of South America, who chewed the bark of

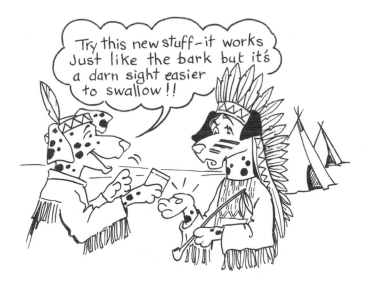

one of the species of willow growing in the forest to relieve pain. It is from the willow that aspirin was originally extracted.

The second use is to reduce the likelihood of the blood forming clots. It works on the platelets, which are tiny disc-like structures that are present in the blood. If you cut yourself, it is the platelets that clump together (aggregate) to form a plug that stops the flow of blood through the broken blood vessels. In stroke due to damage to the brain (infarction), the blood forms a clot inside the artery. This stops the normal flow of blood through the vessel, thereby depriving the brain of oxygen and nutrients. Aspirin stops the platelets sticking to one another and forming a clot. The risk of having another stroke can be reduced by a daily dose of aspirin. Discovering that aspirin is effective in this way was one of the major achievements in medicine in the twentieth century. It has been responsible for saving many thousands of lives, at very little cost and with few side effects.

I am taking aspirin to reduce the chance of my having another stroke. Should my children also take aspirin?

Unless your children have risk factors for stroke other than having you as a parent, there is no reason for them to take aspirin. However, if they do have other problems, such as heart disease or high blood pressure, as well as other members of your family having had a stroke (family history of stroke), our advice would be to take one aspirin a day unless there is a good reason not to.

Will I have to take aspirin for the rest of my life?

If you have had a stroke due to a blood clot forming in an artery and have been put onto aspirin to prevent a further stroke, the answer is probably 'Yes'. It may be that a better treatment will be developed at some time in the future but for the moment aspirin is the safest and most effective treatment available to prevent another stroke. Taking aspirin daily should just become part of your way of life. It is not too serious if you miss the occasional day, because the effects last a long time, but don't stop it altogether without first discussing it with your doctor.

Does aspirin have any side effects?

No drug that works is completely free of side effects. The most common one for aspirin is indigestion due to inflammation of the lining of the stomach. Occasionally, it can cause a stomach ulcer to form – which can bleed, causing anaemia. If you have or have had a stomach ulcer, you should use aspirin with caution. It may be that your doctor will prescribe another drug or else give you an anti-ulcer drug to take at the same time as the aspirin, just to be on the safe side. The benefits of aspirin are so great in preventing further stroke that you and your doctor may decide to take a bit of a risk and have the aspirin anyway and monitor you carefully for side effects.

A few people are allergic to aspirin, either causing them to develop a rash or triggering an asthma attack. It can also cause a major allergic response called *angio-oedema*, in which the tissues of the face and throat swell up, sometimes resulting in difficulty in breathing. If you have a history of aspirin allergy, you should be prescribed a different anti-platelet drug.

You might expect – given the way that aspirin works – that it could cause problems with persistent bleeding if you cut yourself. In fact, this is not a significant problem and is not usually noticeable.

How much aspirin should I take and does it matter which sort I take?

It probably doesn't matter how much aspirin you take, so long as you take some. For the first two weeks after the stroke, when you may be treated with aspirin to help minimise the effects of the stroke, the appropriate dose is 300mg a day. After that time, when the aspirin is being given to prevent another stroke, I [AR] usually reduce the dose to 75mg a day. It is probably as effective as larger doses and is less likely to have side effects. Some doctors prefer to keep people on the 300mg dose whereas others compromise at 150mg. There is no reason for you to take more than 300mg a day. This is a tiny dose compared with that used to treat pain, when it would be usual to take at least 600mg four times a day. You can take it in any form you like.

I think that I'm allergic to aspirin. Is there anything else I can take?

Two newer drugs that are licensed to be used to prevent stroke could be taken as an alternative to aspirin. The first is clopidogrel (Plavix): in a large study of people with a range of diseases caused by 'furring up' of the arteries – including stroke and heart disease – it was as effective as aspirin. It seemed to be safe, with few side effects. The second one is dipyridamole (Persantin or Asasantin), which is an older drug that in early trials did not seem to be useful for stroke prevention. Recently, however, a well-run trial has shown that it is effective, especially when combined with aspirin. The results of this trial suggest that the combination of aspirin and dipyridamole is more effective than aspirin alone. Not all doctors are entirely convinced, and the usual practice is still to prescribe aspirin on its own.

If you are allergic to aspirin, there is probably not much to choose between these two. However, a lot of people have been told that they are allergic to drugs without much evidence that it is true. If there is any serious doubt about your being allergic to aspirin, it may be worth trying it again under carefully supervised conditions, because, if you can tolerate it, the benefits would be great.

I have heard that combining aspirin with a second drug is better than taking aspirin on its own. Is this true?

A trial combining 50mg of aspirin with dipyridamole (Persantin MR 200mg twice a day) produced greater benefit than aspirin used alone. Many doctors in the UK are cautious and are waiting for confirmation of these results before starting their stroke patients on the combination of drugs. Not only are there concerns about whether it really is effective but it would also greatly increase the cost of treatment.

I was already on aspirin when I had my stroke. What next?

If you were already taking aspirin when you had your stroke (or TIA), your doctor should add dipyridamole (Persantin SR) to it. A reasonable alternative would be clopidogrel (Plavix) 75mg daily without the aspirin. The combination of clopidogrel with aspirin is currently being tested and we should have the results of this trial soon. It might prove to be a worthwhile combination, as both drugs work on the platelets in different ways to reduce the risk of blood clots forming.

An alternative that your doctor might consider is the anticoagulant (blood 'thinner') warfarin. This drug has been useful for people who have an irregular heart rhythm due to atrial fibrillation, who have a blood clot in their heart or have the antiphospholipid syndrome. It is not of proven value where the stroke is due to other causes.

I've been advised that I should take warfarin to thin my blood. Is it a good idea?

Warfarin is a drug that slows down the normal clotting mechanism of the blood. It is different from aspirin in that it works on the clotting proteins rather than the platelets. It is very effective at reducing the risk of stroke in people who have atrial fibrillation or blood clots that have formed inside the heart. Taking warfarin will reduce your risk of stroke by about 60%, whereas aspirin reduces the risk by only about 25%. The problem with warfarin, however, is that the dose needs to be very carefully controlled so that the clotting mechanism is not impaired too much. Each individual needs to have the dose adjusted specifically for them. This requires blood tests to monitor what effect the warfarin is having. When you begin taking the drug, your blood will need to be checked every few days. Once the dose is stable, it may only be necessary to repeat the blood test every month. Your requirement for warfarin can be very easily affected by taking other drugs (drug interaction) or doing anything that might affect the function of your liver, such as binge alcohol drinking. If you take warfarin, it is very important to let your doctor or dentist know this before they prescribe anything else. It is also wise to be careful about what you buy over the counter from the chemists; consult the pharmacist to see if there are any possible interactions between warfarin and the drug you want to buy.

The risk associated with taking warfarin is that, if you start bleeding, it will carry on for longer than normal. This doesn't matter if it is just a cut on the skin that you can put a bit of pressure on for a few minutes until it stops, but does matter if the bleeding is internal. So, if you have had a stomach ulcer that has caused problems recently, it is usually unwise to go onto warfarin. Likewise, if you are at significant risk of falling and banging your head, the risk of bleeding on the surface of the brain could outweigh the possible benefit of preventing a stroke. Deciding whether to start warfarin can be quite difficult. The benefits and risks should be discussed with you, and in the end the decision should be left up to you.

I was put on warfarin after my first stroke because I had atrial fibrillation. Now I've had another little stroke and my doctor wants me to take aspirin as well. But the booklet I got from the anticoagulant clinic says the two should not be taken together. What should I do?

The reason why your booklet advises you not to combine warfarin with aspirin is that aspirin can occasionally cause bleeding from the stomach, which, if you are taking an anticoagulant, could be more serious. There is no evidence to show that the combination of aspirin and warfarin is either safe or effective, so it should only be given in exceptional circumstances after very careful consideration by an expert.

My wife had dementia before her stroke and was already quite disabled. Is there really any point her taking aspirin to prevent another stroke?

If it is worth preventing another stroke, it is worth her taking aspirin. It may be that the cause of her dementia was multiple little strokes in the past, so aspirin might prevent it from getting worse by stopping these little strokes from happening.

My cholesterol is not very high but still my doctor wants to start me on treatment to lower it. Do I really need to take yet another tablet?

A research study called the Heart Protection Study has recently shown that nearly everyone who has had a stroke should be taking a statin to reduce the cholesterol. The same argument that we use to explain why the blood pressure should be kept as low as possible also applies to cholesterol. We were not evolved to be able to deal effectively with the very high amounts of animal fats that most of us consume. It looks as though everyone with a total cholesterol of over 3.5mmol/l benefits from a statin, regardless of age. My [AR] practice is therefore to use a statin (usually simvastatin 40mg) for everyone if preventing a stroke within the next two years is a worthwhile objective.

I've read about something called the 'polypill' which if everyone took could dramatically reduce the risk of heart disease and stroke. Where can I get it?

The polypill is at the moment just an idea and is not available. The researchers came up with the idea of combining aspirin, a couple of blood pressure lowering tablets, folic acid and a statin in one tablet. They hypothesise that, if such a pill were taken by everyone over the age of 55, the incidence of stroke and heart disease would be cut by about three-quarters.

They also suggest that such a tablet should be available for the public to buy over the counter rather than requiring it to be prescribed by doctors, so as to reduce the burden on GPs and increase the number of people taking it. There would, however, be some problems with such a strategy. For some people the drugs might actually be dangerous and the cost would be quite high.

The idea is a very interesting one and needs to be tested properly in a medical trial. Until this has been done, our advice is to take the tablets that your doctor recommends and carry on with a healthy active lifestyle.

Now that I have had a stroke can I still use hormone replacement therapy?

My [AR] advice is to stop taking the HRT, as there is some evidence that it might increase the risk of stroke and heart disease. It might well be worth, however, starting a regular calcium supplement to try to keep your bones strong in old age.

Surgery to prevent stroke

I've been told that my carotid artery is narrowed and I should have an operation to unblock it. What does this involve, and what are the risks?

The carotid artery is the blood vessel that carries the blood from the aorta, which is the main artery coming from the heart, to the brain. There is one on each side and they can be felt pulsating either side of the windpipe in your neck. Narrowing of the carotid artery reduces the amount of blood reaching your brain, which, when it becomes severe, can cause a stroke. A fairly straightforward operation, called *carotid endarterectomy*, removes the narrowed portion of vessel, restoring normal blood flow to the brain. The problem is usually identified by performing a *carotid ultrasound* (doppler) and sometimes an *arteriogram*. Research trials in Europe and North America have shown that, if you have had a mild stroke or a TIA and your carotid artery is reduced in diameter by more than 70%, having an operation to clear the narrowing is better than just having medical treatment. If the artery is completely blocked, nothing will be gained by operating. If the narrowing is less than 70%, the risks of surgery outweigh the benefits.

If you agree to the operation, it will be done under a general or a local anaesthetic. A small cut is made over the artery and a temporary tube is inserted above and below the part of the vessel that is narrowed, to allow the brain to continue receiving blood while the blockage is cleared. The damaged part of the artery is then removed and the two cut ends are sewn back together. The whole procedure lasts about half an hour, and if everything has gone smoothly you will probably be home the next day.

The operation is not completely risk free, so the decision to undertake it requires careful consideration. The worry is that the operation itself will result in a stroke. This happens when a piece of the debris that has accumulated inside the artery (causing the narrowing) becomes dislodged and travels up to the brain during the operation. The risk of this occurring is between 3% and 5% when the operation is performed by an experienced surgeon. Otherwise the risks of surgery are small: there may be some local pain and bruising; occasionally, there can be some bleeding around the site of the repair, which may require draining; and wounds can always get infected and require antibiotics.

There is no way of knowing in advance which people will benefit and which will suffer. It is like gambling on the horses: you can know everything about all of the horses, riders and weather conditions and still not be certain of getting rich. No one would choose to have an operation but, if it can greatly reduce your risk of a serious stroke, it is probably a risk worth taking. Find a surgeon who does lots of these operations every year and whom you feel you can trust. Listen carefully to what he or she says and ask whatever questions you want. Give yourself time to think about it and talk to friends and family. Then, if you decide to go ahead with the operation, have it done soon. The more time that passes, the greater the chance of the stroke happening before surgery. In the meantime, keep on taking the aspirin.

My husband may have a carotid angioplasty. What is it?

Instead of opening up the carotid artery and removing the narrowed section of artery surgically (carotid endarterectomy, discussed in the previous answer), in *carotid angioplasty* a narrow tube is put into an artery (usually in the groin) and guided up through the heart and into the carotid. Once the tip is at the level of the narrowed portion of vessel, saline (salt water) is injected into the tube to inflate a small balloon at the end. This dilates (expands) the artery, allowing more blood to pass.

Although this procedure avoids the need for surgery, it still carries the risk of causing a stroke. There has been one study suggesting that it is as effective as surgery but many doctors (especially the surgeons!) still favour operating. It is also not yet known whether surgery and angioplasty are equally effective at preventing stroke in the very long term (years after the procedure has been done). Research is underway to compare the relative advantages and disadvantages of carotid endarterectomy with angioplasty. Until the results are available, unless you are taking part in the trial, it would be wise to opt for the treatment that is of definite proven benefit . . . which is the surgery.

I've got an aneurysm that burst, and I've been advised that it needs surgery to prevent it bleeding again. Should I go ahead?

Definitely. If you don't have the aneurysm repaired, there is a strong possibility that it will bleed again – and you could become seriously ill or die. It is best to have the surgery as soon as possible after the aneurysm has leaked for the first time, because the period of highest risk for rebleeding is within the first two weeks. An aneurysm is part of an artery that has become weakened and has ballooned out as a result of the high pressure normally present inside the vessel. The surgery to repair it will be performed by a specialist neurosurgeon. The operation carries about a 5% risk of causing stroke, but without surgery there is about a 30% chance of your aneurysm rebleeding within a year.

Developing new symptoms

What are the signs I should look out for that would suggest I'm going to have another stroke?

The signs of stroke vary according to which part of the brain is affected. Nearly always a stroke causes problems down one side of the body. The commonest is weakness in an arm or leg, or both. Numbness or tingling can occur. Loss of vision in one eye or loss of vision to either the right or the left side might indicate that a stroke has happened. Problems with language, such as inability to understand what people are saying to you or difficulty in producing the right words or sentences, difficulty co-ordinating your arm or unsteadiness in walking, or suddenly developing double vision are all symptoms that occur with stroke. Almost always the symptoms come on rapidly within a few minutes, although they can come and go over a period of a few hours before staying put.

If you experience any of these symptoms or are worried that others might be due to stroke, seek immediate assistance from your doctor or get up to the local hospital accident and emergency department. Don't be frightened that you may be troubling your doctor unnecessarily. It is far better to be safe than sorry, and anyway it's quite nice for doctors to be able to reassure patients not to worry.

I had an epileptic fit shortly after my stroke. Will I need to stay on the epilepsy drugs for ever?

About 2% of people who have a stroke have an epileptic fit (seizure) on the day of their stroke, and in only half of these does a seizure ever recur. Epilepsy is a condition in which the brain's electrical activity becomes disorganised, producing a variety of symptoms that can range from a twitching finger to a generalised fit associated with loss of consciousness and shaking. There are many causes but if it happened shortly after your stroke and this was confirmed with a brain scan, there is no reason to look for any other reason. A single fit soon after the stroke does not usually need treating with drugs and it would be reasonable to ask your doctor if you can stop them. There is, however, a small risk that you will then have another one, in which case you would have to start taking a tablet to prevent further attacks and stop driving until you had had been free of fits for a year.

My stroke was nine months ago, and I have now had a blackout that my doctor has told me she thinks is likely to have been a fit. Is the stroke the cause, and what should be done?

The most likely cause is the stroke. About 5% of people who have had a stroke, particularly if it was a large one, develop fits in the year after their stroke. The risk of having a fit then falls to about 2% per year after that. Your doctor may want to do some tests to make sure there are no other causes. She may want you to have another brain scan, or an electroencephalogram (EEG), which is a recording of your brain's electrical activity, obtained by placing little electrodes on your scalp. However, if she has a good description of the blackout from someone who saw it, it may not be necessary for you to have the tests.

The treatment is with tablets. There is a wide range of possible drugs she could prescribe, including phenytoin (Epanutin), carbamazepine (Tegretol) and sodium valproate (Epilim). All of them must be used carefully, so that you have just enough of the drug to prevent fits but not cause side effects. The side effects vary according to which drug is used, but all of them can cause nausea and drowsiness. So long as the doses are monitored – usually by blood or saliva tests – it is nearly always possible to find a drug that is effective for you and free of side effects. It is advisable to carry on with the drug for the rest of your life when the fit has developed late after the stroke, because you will always be at risk of further attacks.

I keep having attacks of hiccups, which I never used to get. I've tried holding my breath till I burst but it doesn't work. Do you have any suggestions?

Hiccups have certainly been reported as occurring after strokes affecting the brainstem. Many drugs have been tried, with varying degrees of success, including chlorpromazine, phenytoin, sodium valproate and metoclopramide. All of these carry the risk of side effects, so should be used with caution and only under a doctor's supervision.

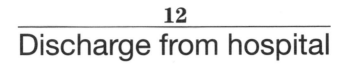

12
Discharge from hospital

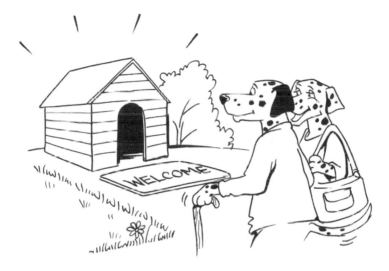

Every hospital should have procedures that have been agreed by a number of agencies, including social services, for the discharge of people from the hospital. The priority should be for you to leave as soon as you are fit enough to do so and when it is safe for you to return home. You should be provided with help to make any necessary arrangements. Planning for your discharge should, ideally, begin as soon as possible in your hospital stay. This may not be feasible early on, however, if there is uncertainty about whether you will be able to return home or will need some form of residential care.

The team of people concerned with your care on the unit or ward should meet regularly to discuss your progress. This meeting will also consider what arrangements will need to be made in order for you to return home. You should be as involved as you are able to be in the discussions and planning for your discharge; your partner, if you have one, and other members of the family should also be consulted and involved. Most teams include a social worker whose job includes linking with community resources. The physiotherapist will be involved in issues concerned with your mobility, and the occupational therapist will advise about any equipment or adaptations to your home. There should also be a named nurse, who will be responsible for ensuring that the most appropriate plan for your discharge is devised and then implemented. In some hospitals there may be a discharge co-ordinator who fulfils this role.

Managing at home

I'm very worried about how I'll manage when I am discharged from hospital. What sort of help can I expect?

Most people feel anxious about how they will manage when they get home. However much preparation for discharge there has been in hospital, you are still likely to be concerned about how you will actually be able to cope. This will be particularly true if you have been left with significant disability. The point at which you are discharged will depend on many factors, not just how much you have recovered. The team looking after you will need to consider the environment you are going back to. For example:

- Will you have to negotiate stairs or can you be set up to live, at least to begin with, on one level?

- Are you going home to live on your own or will there be people around to help?

- How much rehabilitation will be available for you after discharge?

- How much support is there in your area from the social services department?

Once all these things have been considered and discussed with you, a date will be set for you to leave hospital. In many ways the earlier you get back to your own home the better, so long as the right treatment and support are available. It is all very well becoming proficient at getting in and out of a hospital bed or chair and getting to the hospital toilet but the skills needed to do these things may be rather different in your own home.

It may be possible for you to have a home visit with an occupational therapist and others involved (physiotherapist or social worker, for instance) before you are discharged from hospital, to see how you might manage at home and what sort of support and assistance you might need once you are home again. You have to be courageous, though; otherwise, you will never get home. It often proves a lot easier to manage than your imagination would have you believe. And if difficulties are encountered, they may not be all that hard to solve with some perseverance.

What help should I be able to get from the social services department after I leave hospital?

The amount of help available from social services will very much depend on your level of need. A social worker will undertake a Community Care Assessment of you and your needs. They should then, in discussion and partnership with you, produce a care plan that details what care you will receive and who will provide it. Not all of this care is likely to come from the social services department but it is useful for the care plan to provide details of how your needs will be met and by whom. The social worker should also assess any needs that your carer may have for assistance and take these into account in the care plan. A separate Carer Assessment can be provided at the same time as your assessment, or can be requested by your carer if you have had an assessment under the terms of the NHS and Community Care Act. The types of assistance that social services can provide are usually in practical form, such as the provision of home care, meals-on-wheels, day care, help with adaptations and equipment or residential care. There may be some limited help for disabled people with the cost of communication equipment such as telephones or for holidays.

There are some services that the social services department is not likely to provide or to pay for; for example, 24-hour care at home. Nursing care at home is the responsibility of the health authority (health board in Scotland) and is paid for by them. Certain types of equipment, mainly medical or nursing in nature (a specialised bed, for example) would also be unlikely to be provided by social services. If, however, you have enough money to purchase 24-hour care for yourself, the social services department can provide advice and information on this.

In some areas, instead of purchasing services for you, social services will give you the money to buy them yourself, through a scheme called Direct Payments; or you can have a mix of provision by social services and Direct Payments. The money must be used to buy care services; it cannot be used for ordinary household expenses. There are particular criteria for Direct Payments, so it is best to discuss the possibility with your social services department. In any case, they should give you advice and information on how to use the payments to purchase such care.

Most social services departments have eligibility criteria to decide what services they will provide, assistance being given to those most in need. There are likely to be charges for many, if not all, of the services that you receive at home, so there will also be a financial assessment to determine how much you can contribute to the cost of any care services that are provided.

Where can I find out about voluntary organisations that might be able to help me after I have left hospital?

There should be some leaflets available in your ward, explaining what the local voluntary organisations offer. If not, contact The Stroke Association or Different Strokes (details in Appendix 1) and they will be able to put you in touch with your local group. Other useful organisations include Chest, Heart & Stroke Scotland, Northern Ireland Chest, Heart & Stroke Association, and Speakability (addresses in Appendix 1).

My mother still has lots of problems after her stroke. She has difficulty walking and is very unsteady on her feet, and she still gets a bit confused. I don't think she is ready to go home and think that she should go into a nursing home. But she refuses. How can I make her change her mind?

Recovery from stroke can take a long time and people can continue to improve for many months. Motivation to work towards recovery can vary, however, and a positive attitude is often vital. If your mother is forced to go into a care home against her wishes, she may lose hope and fail to continue to improve. But if she is presented with a challenge, such as recovering enough to go home, she may work hard towards this aim. If she doesn't recover enough to be able to return home, or returns home but cannot cope, alternative arrangements may have to be made. Your mother might accept this at that point, however, because she has had the chance to try to get home or even to be at home. If she is not given the chance to try, she may be very resentful or have very unrealistic views about 'if only . . .'.

Generally speaking, it is not possible to force people to change their minds, but they may do so gradually over a period of time. As an adult, your mother should be able to take her own decisions, and these should be respected even though you may be worried about her safety. If her degree of confusion is very great, you may need to discuss with members of the hospital team whether she is able to take such decisions. If necessary, they will involve a psychiatrist to assess her capacity to make decisions.

Whether your mother should return home is a slightly different question, and in this you and she need to be guided by the views of the team who have been caring for her. They will have formed views about whether your mother is likely to be able to manage at home and will discuss these with you both. It may be that a further period of treatment in a rehabilitation centre can be arranged to allow for a longer recovery period. It may also be that your mother would agree to go into a care home temporarily to continue with her rehabilitation. It is possible, however, that you may need to find a more specialised nursing home that has a focus on rehabilitation. Such a care home could continue, perhaps, to provide therapy or access to local rehabilitation facilities for your mother.

I'm hoping to go home soon. Should I arrange to see a social worker?

It could be helpful to arrange to see a social worker in order to discuss what types of help you might obtain when you return home. The social worker should be able to give you advice and information about the range of services that might be available. However, if the hospital is not in the area where you live, the social worker may have to contact social services in that area in order to obtain information from them (social workers don't know everything about everywhere!). The social worker may be involved in helping to arrange for services to help you at home, and to establish the care plan for your discharge from hospital – in which case you should probably see them on a regular basis before you leave the hospital.

If you are not going to be able to return home and are considering a care home, it would be useful to see a social worker for advice and information. If you will need help to pay for part or all of this type of care, it is essential to see a social worker, as the arrangements will have to be made through your local authority's social services department.

Social workers can also help with discussions about illness and disability. They are not just involved in practical solutions, and may also provide some help with relationship and emotional problems. Many social workers have had some training in counselling, but, because they often have a heavy workload, they may be able to offer counselling only while you are in hospital.

My father is going to need a lot of help when he goes home. Should I give up work to look after him?

This is a difficult decision to take and requires both you and your father, and even other family members, to be involved in making it. You will need to consider your financial position:

- Can you afford to give up work?

- What is the likely effect on your family (if you have one) and what are their views about this matter?

- Do you have room for your father to live with you without causing overcrowding in your home, or would you need to move?

Other questions to be considered are those concerning your relationship:

- Is it a strong relationship?

- Could it withstand the possible rigours of caring?

- Could you provide personal, even intimate, care to your father?

- Could you care for him for a long time, perhaps indefinitely?

- What sources of help might be available to you to help you to care, especially if over a long period?

- What is the view of your employer and colleagues – could you take compassionate leave or work part-time for a while?

- What will be your chances of being able to return to work after caring for your father?

It could be helpful to discuss these issues with somebody outside the family before reaching a final decision. A social worker or counsellor may be able to help you (and perhaps your family) to consider the many different aspects of this issue and to reach a decision that is the right one for you, your father and anyone else concerned.

I'd really like to get out of hospital but realise that I'm not quite well enough to go home yet. Is there a sort of half-way house?

It is usually possible to arrange a period of care or convalescence in a care home (with or without nursing care) – or even a hotel – after discharge, although you would probably have to pay for this yourself. (Some charities can occasionally help: your local Citizens Advice Bureau may be able to provide information on those in your area that might assist; or consult *A Guide to Grants for People in Need* in your local library.)

Whether it is wise to have convalescence is another matter. Going home needs careful planning, sometimes requiring a complex package of care to be started from the day you leave hospital. This can be more difficult to organise if you go off to convalescence first. In addition, it may well be important to continue with your rehabilitation after discharge and it is unlikely that you would get the appropriate treatment in a care home unless it was a home that specialised in rehabilitation (not very commonly found). It might be better to get yourself established at home for a few weeks first and then think about a holiday.

Moving in with the family

I am considering having my mother to come and live with me but my husband and children are not very keen. What should I do?

This is a difficult one to answer. Some people take decisions in a hurry because they believe it is the right thing to do, or because they feel a duty to do so, or because they feel some pressure on them to make a decision quickly. Not everyone is able to care for a relative, especially if they are really quite dependent, but sometimes it is hard to recognise or acknowledge this. If your family are not keen on the idea, it may be better not to enter an arrangement that could become very difficult and antagonistic, and create lasting tension in the family. The decision must be one that everyone feels as comfortable as possible with: you, your family, your mother and perhaps also the wider family.

Before you make a final decision, it is a good idea to seek advice and information from, say, a social worker or a support group such as Carers UK. A social worker or counsellor may be able to help you (and perhaps your family) to consider the many factors involved in caring for someone and to reach a decision that is the right one for you and your family. Thinking carefully about the question and considering as many of the different angles as possible over a period of time is usually better than rushing into a decision because you feel you ought to do so. A rushed, incorrect decision may not be easy to put right later.

I'm having my mother to come and live with me. She had a big stroke and is going to need a lot of looking after. But I have children at home and I'm just not sure how I'm going to give her all the attention she needs. Will I be allowed to leave her on her own for short periods?

You will be taking on a big job and it's sensible to think through carefully exactly what it is going to involve, not just from you but also from everyone else in the family. Remember that probably none of the possible solutions for the care of your mother is going to be perfect. Presumably the option of her going back to her own home has been ruled out because the care she needs cannot all be provided by the social services and the family. The alternative of a nursing home would have the advantages of taking the load of providing physical care off you, giving you more time to be with her socially. The disadvantages, however, can often be great. Living with a lot of people you don't know, and may never have wanted to know, many of whom will be severely physically or mentally disabled, is trying. Most of us fight to keep out of institutions all our lives (hospitals, prisons, the army) because we recognise that institutional life restricts our freedom.

You have made the decision to have your mother to live with you. The care you provide will almost certainly be better than that given elsewhere, because it will be given with love. But if you set out thinking you can do everything that she wants and be there all the time to tend to her needs, you are bound to fail. You would get physically and emotionally exhausted and probably end up taking it out on the rest of your family. We assume that you are not a saint!

Set out clearly with your mother in advance what you will be able to do for her and what the limits are. Of course, you may have to go out and leave her on her own. Even if she was in a nursing home, she would be spending quite large parts of the day and most of the night on her own. What is the worst that can happen? She might have another stroke or fall out of her chair and break her hip. How would you have prevented either of those things happening if you had been in the kitchen? In neither instance would the outcome be any different whether you were there to help in five minutes or four hours. Of course, you don't want to leave her distressed on her own for four hours if you don't have to, but if the alternative is nursing home care it may not be such a big price to pay.

In many parts of the country there is some sort of 'sitting service' (e.g. Crossroads or local voluntary groups) whereby someone will come in for a few hours each week to allow carers to go out. Another possibility would be for your mother to go to a day centre for a day or two a week. Not only would this give you some time for yourself but would also give your mother an opportunity to meet other people. The local social services department should have information about what is available in your area.

Moving into sheltered housing

I don't think I'll be able to cope on my own back home, but I don't really need to go into a care home. How about sheltered housing?

Sheltered housing – which may be flats, houses, maisonettes or bungalows – usually has an on-site warden who can help the tenants, but that is often the limit of the assistance provided. The warden may make regular contact with people to check that they are okay or they may be available to summon help if people need urgent assistance.

Sheltered accommodation may be owned and run by the local authority, by housing associations or by voluntary organisations or charities, usually on a rented basis. In some of the newer developments, units can be purchased and the property sold back when it is no longer required. Be careful to check out service charges, though; they can sometimes rise sharply over the years.

Some local authority sheltered housing may be adapted for disabled people but there will probably be a waiting list for places. A small number of developments, usually called 'very special sheltered housing', may also provide residential or nursing home care on the same site so that if someone eventually needs that type of care they don't necessarily have to move very far to receive it. Housing with care schemes may also exist and provide higher levels of help in the home to the tenants. Your local authority's housing department or advice services should be able to provide advice and information on what is available in your area.

Before you consider moving into sheltered accommodation, think hard about what advantages it would offer. The wardens do not provide any physical care. They are really only there to act as a good neighbour and to respond if there is an emergency. You could be moving away from your friends and neighbours to a housing complex occupied mainly or solely by older people. As well as which, wardens vary. Many are extremely helpful but there are also those who don't really want to be bothered. If you call for help in the middle of the night more than a few times, they may well insist that you leave and go into residential care.

If you have to move anyway because you are in unsuitable accommodation, sheltered housing is probably the right option. But think about staying put and perhaps getting an alarm that you wear round your neck or on your wrist and can press if you are in trouble. In some areas you must have someone who agrees to respond to emergencies, but in many districts the local authority has a central control system that will send out one of their staff if no one else is available.

Moving into a care home

The official names of residential and nursing homes are now 'care home' and 'care home (nursing)'. For simplicity, though, we refer to them here as care homes (whether residential or nursing) and nursing homes if we mean only homes that provide nursing care.

I am thinking of going into a care home. How do I choose one, and who would pay?

You will usually be helped to arrange for care in a nursing or residential home through the hospital stroke team and your local social services department. If you have sufficient long-term finance, of course you can approach a private nursing home, for example, and make your own arrangements with them. However, such care homes typically cost upwards of £450 a week, and in some areas costs are much higher, so many people need help to pay for a place. If this is the case for you, you will need to contact your local social services department about this. It is also possible that they will not be able to pay the full cost of the home, so any shortfall would have to be made up by you or your family. Care for nursing/medical needs should be free in nursing homes, however, so the charges would only be for your personal care and accommodation. In some homes, these charges may still be quite high, however, and are likely to increase every year. It may be possible to get help for payments through charities, although there are very few that provide such help over the long term.

You may already be in touch with a social worker in the hospital; if you are not, ask the ward/unit staff to help you to make contact. The social worker should provide advice and information about the different homes in your area. If at all possible, visit a few homes in order to discuss with the owners/managers what your requirements are likely to be and to find the one that will suit your needs best. If you are not able to visit them yourself, ask someone who knows you well, perhaps your partner or another member of the family, to help. If possible, you should also visit the home before moving in: this will become your home and it is important to make sure it is the right place for you. Some homes will arrange for you to stay for a short time in order to be sure that you will be happy there. You could treat it as a holiday while you make up your mind.

If you need help with the funding of a place in a home, the social worker will assess your needs for care. (If you remain in your own home, any needs that your partner might have as a carer should also be taken into account.) There will also be a financial assessment (means-test) of your abilities to contribute towards the cost of the care. Once these assessments have taken place, however, it should be possible to arrange for admission to the home fairly quickly. In a nursing home, you should only be expected to pay for personal care/board and lodging costs if you have established long-term medical or nursing needs (which should be met by the NHS). In such cases, your contribution would be towards the personal/accommodation costs of your care. If your placement is financially supported by a local council, they should pay for all the costs; the local primary care trust will then pay the council for your nursing care, whilst you contribute towards the personal care and accommodation costs.

Although it will take some time for you to settle into the home, and for you to get used to this change, it may make your relationships with your partner and family easier in the long term. In some cases you may be able to have visits home, or your partner may be able to stay overnight in the home (although there is likely to be a charge for this).

Do I have to go into a home near where I live or can I move to a home nearer my daughter?

If you are paying for a place in a home, you can decide where that home is. If, on the other hand, you are receiving help from social services to pay for a place, it will depend on the cost involved. Social services can pay for places in homes in areas other than the one you live in, but only up to a certain level of payment (usually what they would pay in your home area). This might not present a problem, as the costs in the two areas may be the same, or the home near your daughter might be willing to accept a slightly lower fee. Your family or a charity might be willing to pay the difference in cost, and enter into an arrangement with social services about this, called a Third Party Agreement. Remember, however, that this type of commitment may be open ended and long term, and it may not be possible or advisable for your family to pay over a lengthy period. In nursing homes, medical and nursing costs should be free, but the cost of personal care and accommodation over a lengthy period can still be substantial. In addition, you also need to decide whether in the longer term you would like to be nearer to your daughter or to stay closer to friends and former neighbours so that they can visit you easily.

What is the difference between a nursing home and a residential home?

Both types of home are subject to the provisions of the Registered Homes Act 1984, which set out requirements for all homes with more than three residents to be registered with either the health authority (health board in Scotland) – for nursing homes – or the local authority – for residential homes. This is how the homes obtain their registration and, in a sense, their licence to operate, as home owners have to establish that they have (and continue to have) sufficient facilities, accommodation, equipment and staff to run such a home. Some homes are run privately as businesses, some are run by voluntary organisations or charities on a not-for-profit basis, and a few residential homes are owned and run by the local authority.

The principal differences between residential and nursing homes are in the level of care provision and staffing. Nursing homes must, by law, have at least one trained and registered nurse on the premises 24 hours a day. Some residential homes also provide this but they are not legally required to do so. There is also likely to be some specialised equipment available in nursing homes to cater for the medical and nursing needs of the residents, and some very specialised homes may have on-site therapy and rehabilitation services. There are a growing number of dual-registered homes – homes that provide both nursing and residential care: if someone who has been receiving residential care (for lesser care needs) eventually requires nursing level care, they do not have to move to another home for that extra care.

Changes in the registration system mean that care homes are registered and inspected by one authority rather than the previous system of either health or social services, depending on the type of home. Registration now rests with the Commission for Social Care Inspection (CSSI), set up by the Government to oversee the provision of care in both residential and nursing homes.

I'm only 52 years old and have had a big stroke. I can't look after myself any more but I don't want to go into a home full of old people. Will I be able to find anything appropriate?

Although by far the largest number of homes is for older people, there are also specialist homes that cater for younger disabled people. There are fewer of these, however, and some of them have waiting lists. It will also depend on the level of your need – some homes provide very specialist care and are therefore very expensive if you don't actually need this. As you have had a major stroke, however, it is perhaps more likely that you will need care in a specialised nursing home that can offer special facilities, including some therapy and work on rehabilitation. Some organisations, such as the John Groom's Association or the Leonard Cheshire homes, provide care homes especially for disabled people, so you should make contact with them (details in Appendix 1). The on-going costs of any nursing/medical needs you have in the nursing home should be met by the NHS, so you would contribute only towards the cost of personal care and accommodation.

Your local support group (Different Strokes – an organisation specifically for younger people who have had strokes; The Stroke Association; Chest, Heart & Stroke Scotland; Northern Ireland Chest, Heart & Stroke Association) should be able to provide you with information about what homes might be available and what they might offer you. The local registration unit for nursing and residential homes can also provide advice and information; they can also let you see copies of their inspection reports on the homes, as these are available to the public. The hospital social worker may also be able to help with this. So it should be possible for you to find something to suit your needs.

Some assistance may also be possible through the Independent Living (1993) Fund. This fund gives grants to help people with severe impairments to pay for care services in their own homes. To qualify, a person must be aged between 16 and 66, expect to live in the community for at least six months, be receiving the highest rate of the care component of the Disability Living Allowance and have a reduced amount of capital (e.g. savings of less than £18,500 in 2004; this excludes the value of any property but includes the value of any capital that a partner may have). There are also requirements about the amount of services or Direct Payments that the person is receiving from social services and the need for additional services from elsewhere. There is a maximum available to assist someone, which is a combined amount from the Independent Living Fund and the social services department. Further details can be obtained from your local social services department or from the Independent Living Fund (contact details in Appendix 1).

A further scheme known as Direct Payments may also be relevant for you. This cash payment scheme is generally intended to help people with needs relating to disabling conditions, and has been extended to include older people with care needs. In this situation, following assessment, discussion and planning with social services, you may be eligible for an amount of money each week, which you can then use to buy in the care you need at home, rather than have the services arranged by the local authority. Such an arrangement may give you much greater control and independence over your circumstances although there are certain conditions. The scheme means that you act as employer of the individuals who provide the care, which may be more than you either wish or are able to do. Further details about this scheme should be available from your local social services office (see your telephone directory for contact details).

Miscellaneous

Will I need to come up to the out-patients department after discharge?

This will vary according to how services are organised in your area. Your doctor may well want to see you at least once after your discharge from hospital, to make sure that all the arrangements are working as expected and that everything is being done to reduce your risk of further stroke. And, once you have left hospital, you may realise that there are questions you wanted to ask. However, if you have a good GP, he or she may well be happy to take over the supervision of your medical care once you are home. You should be clear when you leave the hospital what the arrangements are for follow-up. If in doubt, ask. In particular, it is important to be clear what you need to do about your medication. The hospital will usually give you only a week or two's supply of tablets, even if they want you to continue with them long term. They will probably expect you to get further supplies from your GP. If you do need to go to the out-patient clinic, the hospital should be able to organise an ambulance or taxi for you and a carer if it would be difficult for you to get there any other way.

I don't like my GP and don't think that, now I've had a stroke, he will give me the amount of attention I need. Can I change, and how do I find a good one?

You are free to change your GP any time you wish. All you need to do is find one who is happy to take you on. The best way to choose a new GP is to ask local friends and neighbours for the names of doctors they like. If that is difficult, you can get the names of local GPs from the local health authority (health board in Scotland), whose number will be in the phone book. You don't have to explain to your old doctor why you are changing. An alternative to changing might be to see your old GP and explain your concerns to him. It may be that, now you have something wrong that is going to need his help, he will be much better than you expect.

I wasn't at all happy with the care I got in hospital. How do I complain?

You should ask to see your consultant or the ward manager to voice your concerns. If you are still unsatisfied, write to the chief executive of the hospital and ask him or her to make enquiries on your behalf. If you are still unhappy with the reply, you can ask for an independent review of your case. This can be a bit slow but is worth doing if you feel strongly that there are fundamental problems with the care given. Even though it may be too late to put right what happened to you, it is important to make sure that it doesn't happen to anyone else. Don't be shy to complain. Unfortunately, it is true that one of the best ways to change things in the health service is to make a complaint. Try to make your complaint as soon as possible after the event. (Your local health authority/health board should be able to give you advice about how to do this.) Don't worry that it will adversely affect your care because it won't. The sooner it's dealt with, the more chance that the error won't be repeated.

On the other hand, if you were happy with the treatment you received, it really helps staff morale if you say so!

13
Relationships

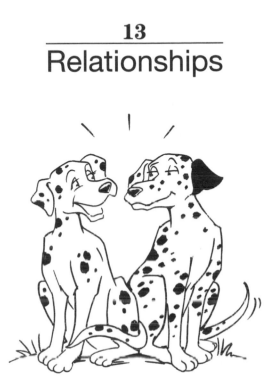

As we have seen, stroke is an illness that can have different effects, depending on the part of the brain that has been injured and the extent of the damage that has occurred. Any on-going problem of circulation and heart disease may also have continuing effects, which can be psychological as well as physical.

It is not unusual for people who have had a stroke to experience depression after it and for there to be some change in their personality. Psychological problems, including feeling anxious, very tired or depressed, and difficulty with concentrating, remembering and making decisions and plans may also occur. Changes in emotional state can also be fairly common; for example, the individual can show *emotionalism* and be irritable and

easily upset and tearful, or seem to be less interested in everyday
life than before. Whether this is likely to continue to be the case
depends on the extent of the damage from the stroke and the
degree of recovery possible.

In addition, it may take some time for relationships to settle
down following the stroke. A major illness is a source of worry
and concern for everybody involved, and it can take many
months for everyone to get used to what has happened and to
adjust to the changes that the illness has produced. Being able to
talk to each other about these effects can be very important in
helping the process of restoring stability. Sometimes it can be
useful to have help with this, perhaps through contact with a
counsellor or social worker.

Sexual matters

**Can my partner and I resume our sex life? I'm really
frightened that he'll have another stroke in the middle
of it.**

He is no more likely to have another stroke in the middle of
making love than at any other time. However, if his stroke was
due to a brain haemorrhage (bleeding into the brain) rather than
an infarct (an area of cell death), it is sensible not to have sex for
the first couple of weeks after the stroke, because his blood
pressure may rise at the time of the orgasm. After the first few
weeks it might actually be more stressful, and therefore harmful,
not to have sex. An active love life is also quite a good way of
getting exercise and keeping the heart fit!

**We always had such a happy sex life before my partner's
stroke. Now that she has to have a urinary catheter, I'm
worried that we won't be able to have sex any more.**

There is no reason why, if you have had a happy sexual
relationship with your partner in the past, this should not be

possible in the future. Whatever the difficulties, you must talk about them together and share the problem. The Outsiders organisation has a sex and disability helpline: it can give you advice over the phone or put you in touch with a local counsellor/therapist if you would prefer this (for contact details see Appendix 1). Many organisations that counsel couples also provide psychosexual counselling.

There are simple methods for both men and women to have sexual intercourse even with a catheter in place, and you should not see this as a bar to continuing to have a happy sexual relationship with your partner. The important thing is to share the problem and the solutions together.

When I was on holiday abroad, a doctor told me that under no circumstances must I have an orgasm, even by masturbation, because it could set off another stroke. I'm only 24 years old. Will I ever be able to enjoy sex again?

There are some unbelievably ignorant doctors around, and not just abroad! First, it is not possible for men to completely avoid orgasms, as they often happen during sleep. Secondly, there is absolutely no evidence that stroke can be precipitated by orgasm unless it was about to happen anyway. It is a normal body function, and getting frustrated by having all sexual activity banned is more likely to do harm than good.

If your stroke was due to bleeding from an aneurysm (a weak spot in one of your arteries) that had not yet been repaired (clipped), there might be a slightly increased risk of stroke during sex; this would be an extremely rare situation, though, as nearly everyone would have the aneurysm clipped shortly after the first bleed.

I've had difficulty getting an erection since I came out of hospital. Would it be safe for me to use Viagra?

Viagra is a relatively new drug that has proved highly effective for men who have difficulty in getting erections and achieving orgasm. Because it is new, there is not much evidence to show whether it is safe following stroke. Stroke is one of the conditions listed as possibly being unsafe ('contra-indicated'), so Viagra cannot be recommended at least in the early stages after a stroke. If there is a risk from using the drug after stroke, it would be greatest in the first few weeks or months. Beyond that time you may feel that it is worth a try, but you must understand that the manufacturer won't take any responsibility if anything goes wrong. Viagra is not available on the NHS for people with impotence following stroke, so you would have to pay for it yourself.

Are there any other treatments available for impotence?

The first thing to do is find out why you have difficulty getting an erection. There are many reasons, both physical and psychological. If the simple causes have been ruled out, there are products that can be used safely after stroke. One is an injection into the penis, which you give yourself just before making love, that produces a temporary erection. It may sound awful but many men use it regularly with great success. A newer product, Aloprostadil, is a preparation containing prostaglandin, which is a naturally occurring substance that causes inflammation; it is inserted into the urethra (the hole at the end of the penis), and is said to be as effective as the injection and more acceptable for some people.

If these treatments are unsuccessful or unsuitable, it is possible to have an operation to insert into the penis a device that can be inflated to produce an erection. None of these treatments is quite as bad as they might sound! The first step is to discuss the possible options with your GP, who can refer you on to a specialist at the hospital. Talking about it does not commit you to following any particular path. It is worth taking your partner along with you, as he or she will need to be a willing participant in any treatment.

The Sexual Dysfunction Association may also be able to offer help and advice (contact details in Appendix 1).

**I find making love difficult because I just can't move
enough. What can you recommend?**

If you have paralysis after a stroke, making love can be a major
test of ingenuity but one that can be fun to try to overcome. Most
couples who have been together for some time have sex using
only a small range of positions. These may well not be feasible
after your stroke, and it will be a question of trial and error
finding one that suits both of you. If you used to be on top, try
getting your partner to swap round. Side-lying positions can be
comfortable and not require much physical exertion.

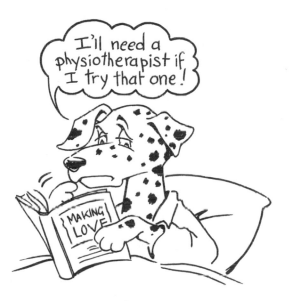

There are lots of books and videos that illustrate the various
options. Some of their suggestions are nigh on impossible, even
for the most physically agile of couples, but they may give you
some ideas. Whatever you try can't do you any harm, except that
you might die laughing! Your physiotherapist should be able to
give you some advice on what might suit you best.

I never used to have problems having an orgasm when I made love to my husband but since my stroke I just don't seem to manage it any more. Why is this?

The reasons why you might be having difficulty could be physical or psychological, or both. It is very common to lose interest in sex after a stroke. You are quite likely to be more tired at the end of the day than you used to be, partly as a direct result of the stroke and partly because you may be having to make much more of an effort just to do the basic physical tasks of looking after yourself and your family.

If all you want to do when you get to bed is to go to sleep, sex won't get much of a look in. Try making love in the morning when you first wake up. Depression or low mood is very common after stroke and is often accompanied by a loss of sexual appetite. Anxiety about whether sex might cause you to have another stroke could be playing a part. If you have difficulty moving in bed while making love, that might affect your ability to have an orgasm. It can also be difficult to come to terms with your own view of yourself – people sometimes feel that their body is damaged and ugly. Sex can become a vicious circle where you don't achieve climax, which adds to your anxiety the next time around. Start by getting to know each other again, just being physically close without attempting to reach orgasm. Then one day, when you are least expecting it, it'll happen.

Some of the drugs that are used to treat high blood pressure (hypertension) can affect sexual function in men and women. If this is a possibility, get your doctor to prescribe one of the many alternatives to find one that doesn't have this side effect. If your stroke affected sensation and caused numbness down one side or part of one side of your body, it is possible that you are just less sensitive than you used to be. It may well be that this will recover with time. If the stroke affected your frontal lobe, this could interfere with normal sexual function. This too may improve over time.

Often the cause of the problem is due to a combination of several of these factors. Your specialist or GP will be able to help you identify what the problem might be. Another option would be to discuss it with a sex therapist, who will have wide experience of the sorts of ways that you might be helped.

Is anal sex more dangerous after stroke than other types of sex?

Anal sex is not associated with any particular problems after stroke, either homosexual or heterosexual.

When my husband makes love to me, it is painful and so I no longer enjoy it. Is this due to the stroke?

This is unlikely to be due to your stroke. It would be worth mentioning the problem to your doctor, as it may be simple to remedy. A common cause of painful sex for women after the menopause is vaginal dryness due to lack of the secretions. Using a vaginal lubricant such as K-Y jelly or treatment with oestrogen creams or hormone replacement therapy (HRT) might be appropriate.

Family planning

I want to have another baby. Will it be safe for me to do so after my stroke?

If your stroke was the result of *antiphospholipid syndrome*, this can also result in difficulties with carrying a baby until full term. It is important that all the necessary tests have been done to try to explain why you had the stroke in the first place. Only once this has been done would it be wise to try to have another baby.

If your stroke was originally due to a subarachnoid haemor- rhage resulting from an aneurysm that had not been repaired, it might be wise to have the aneurysm treated first. If this can't be done, your obstetrician would probably recommend that you have a caesarean because of the worry about causing the aneurysm to leak again if you were to have a vaginal delivery.

If your stroke was not the result of either of these two circumstances, there is no reason why it should be any more difficult for
you to conceive or continue with a normal pregnancy and give
birth to a normal baby.

**What sort of contraception should I use now that I've had
a stroke?**

You should not use the combined oestrogen/progesterone pill,
because of the slightly increased risk of causing stroke. Any of
the other methods could be used, including the progesterone-only
pill. Discuss with your partner and your GP or family planning
clinic what would suit you best.

Help for family carers

**I've given up everything to look after my husband but I
don't think he appreciates it. I'm so fed up and tired. I've
even come close to hitting him and often I'll ignore him
even when I know he needs help. I feel terrible but I can't
stand him any longer. Can anyone help?**

Stroke is an illness that affects not only the individual but also
everyone involved with that person. Families, and especially
partners, are likely to be deeply affected too. It is important that
this is recognised from early on in the illness and that you have
the opportunity to obtain appropriate information and support.
You may also need practical help to manage at home, particularly
if your partner has a number of care needs following the recovery
phase. It is quite likely that the stroke happened very suddenly,
without warning. This can make it difficult to get used to the new
situation and may mean that some hopes and expectations for the
future have had to be changed or put on hold. This can be
difficult to accept, particularly if the changes are major and there
is still uncertainty about the future.

Caring for someone full time, especially if it was not

anticipated, can be a difficult and tiring job. It may also be the case, of course, that you have had to change your lifestyle and routines, perhaps giving up work to look after your husband. This can be stressful, and at times it can seem very lonely and isolated, especially if it seems that he does not appreciate the extent of your help. It is important not to 'bottle up' such feelings and let them get on top of you, and that you find someone you trust with whom you can discuss them. This may be a close friend or a relative, or it may be a social worker or counsellor.

It is crucial that you do not try to carry on regardless, for feelings of pressure and resentment can reach a point where you may hurt your husband, either physically or psychologically. Neglect of his care needs can also be harmful in the longer term and lead to other health problems. No doubt this would be likely to be very distressing for both of you, so if you find yourself feeling this way, do not hesitate to ask for help.

I don't seem to be able to do anything right any more. I really try hard to please my partner but all he does is complain. Can I get any help?

Stroke is an illness that affects both the individual and the whole family. Partners are perhaps especially likely to be distressed by the illness and its effects – not just on the person but on everyone close to them. This should be acknowledged from the beginning of the illness and it is essential that you get appropriate information and support. You may also need practical assistance to help you manage at home, as we have seen in Chapter 12. It can take a long time to get used to the stroke and its effects, and for everyone to adjust to what has happened. Your partner may be frustrated at his seeming lack of progress, wanting to recover as quickly as possible, and that frustration may lead to annoyance and complaints that are even directed at you.

It is important that you find time for yourself every so often. Caring for someone can be very tiring, particularly if it involves a lot of physical tasks (such as lifting and moving them). It can be stressful, and can make you feel very lonely and isolated if your partner does not seem to appreciate what you are doing. It can help to have a break from each other and recharge your batteries every so often. This may be on a regular basis, perhaps once a week, to give you the chance to do something different, or even catch up on some sleep. Day care may be provided in a day hospital or rehabilitation unit if your partner needs on-going treatment or therapy. For details about how to gain access to a hospital-based day unit, ask someone from the team who have been treating your partner, or contact your family GP for details. The Health Information Service may also have details about this (see Appendix 1 for contact details).

Day care may also be provided in a day centre run by social services or a voluntary organisation. This may be through a stroke club in your area, or by some other organisation such as Age Concern locally. There is likely to be a charge for attending a day centre, and perhaps also for transport if this is needed to take your partner to and from a centre. Charges vary between areas, but generally will be based on a financial assessment of your partner's ability to contribute towards the cost of the care provided. In some areas there is a lot of demand for places; entry to such centres is through the social services department, who can arrange for an assessment of your partner's needs (if this did not happen while he was in hospital).

In many areas there are now carers' support groups. These are groups that are especially for relatives and friends who are caring for ill and disabled people at home. A national organisation that supports carers with local groups or projects is Carers UK (contact details, including their website, in Appendix 1). Some areas have local stroke clubs, which provide advice and support for people who have had strokes and their carers. There may also be meetings arranged by health professionals in your area, or by The Stroke Association or Different Strokes (an organisation specifically for younger people who have had strokes). Sharing experiences with other people whose situations are similar to yours can be very helpful. You may prefer to join a specialised group, perhaps for people who have had strokes and their families, or a more general one for carers as a whole. It is important to find something that best suits your needs. To find out more about local carer groups and what might be available in your area, contact your local stroke team, your family GP or the Health Information Service (see Appendix 1 for this and other useful contacts).

A neighbour has suggested that we get some respite care for my partner. What is this, and how can I arrange for it?

Respite care is where someone else looks after your partner while you have a break. This break can be a couple of hours a week or perhaps a week or a fortnight from time to time. For the longer periods, either you go away or, perhaps more likely, your partner goes into a hospital or care home to be looked after while you have a break. Relatives or friends might come into your home and look after your partner while you are away, or you both might prefer a formal arrangement with a private agency (domiciliary or nursing care) to provide a live-in carer, or series of carers.

If your finances are limited, it may be possible for the social services department to help with the cost, but you and your partner will need to be assessed by them for your eligibility for this and also to determine how much you (jointly) can pay towards the cost of such care. (The social services department is not required to purchase nursing care for people in their own homes; this is paid for by the health service, so possible assistance with this type of care would need to be discussed with the specialist stroke team or your family GP.)

Respite care for longer or regular periods away from home will usually be arranged through your GP or the hospital stroke team if your partner needs regular in-patient treatment or re-assessment, or for a medical condition to be stabilised. More usually, however, it is likely to be provided through your local social services department. If money is no object, you can approach a private nursing home, for example, and make your own arrangements with them. Such homes typically cost upwards of £450 a week, however, and in some places fees are much higher (and of course will increase annually). Many people therefore need help to fund places in homes, even on a short-term basis, and you should then contact your local social services department about this. The social services department will provide advice and information about the different homes in your area. As with paying for care at home, if you need help with the funding of a temporary place in a home, your partner's needs (for care and respite) will be assessed, and your needs as a carer will be taken into account. There will also be a financial assessment of your abilities to contribute towards the cost of the care. As we have seen in Chapter 12, you should only contribute towards the personal and accommodation costs of the nursing home, as the costs of nursing and medical needs should be met by the NHS. If you meet the social services criteria, it may be possible to arrange for regular respite periods. This will probably make caring for your partner easier to manage, and may ease any strain on your relationship with each other. He might also welcome a break from you!

What advice can you give me to protect my own health and well-being as a carer?

Caring for someone with a disability can be a tiring and sometimes thankless task. It can also take its toll on the physical and psychological health of the carer. Depression, anxiety and physical disease are much more common among carers than the general public as a whole. If at all possible, don't take on the whole responsibility yourself. Find others to share it with you. Talk to relatives and friends to see if they can offer some help. Use the services that the local authority and the health services have available, even if at first you think you can manage without them. Plan regular breaks. If your partner cannot be left alone, see if a member of the family will come and take over your role for a week or two. If not, ask social services to arrange a period of respite care in a residential or nursing home. See if there is a local branch of Crossroads (address in Appendix 1), an organisation that can provide a sitting service for perhaps a few hours a week, while you go out to see friends, go shopping or even just go to sleep. In some areas, Crossroads can also supply live-in carers to cover periods when you want to go away.

If you are beginning to feel the strain, talk to your GP, who can either offer direct help or put you in touch with a counsellor.

There may also be a local carers' group in your area. It can be really helpful to meet with other people in a similar situation, and they may have found solutions to the problems that you have been struggling with.

My mother is determined to go home again after her stroke, even though she needs a lot of help. She refuses to have any of the professional help that has been offered, saying that I can do it all for her. I love her very much, but over the last few years she has become increasingly demanding and she is taking over my life completely. I can't refuse her and don't know what to do.

Now is the time to be strong and stand up for yourself. Your mother has every right to insist on going home, but she does not have the right to demand that you give up your life for her. It would be helpful to talk to your doctor about it and get his or her support for you in setting up some sort of contract between you and your mother.

Try to arrange a meeting with the doctor, your mother and yourself to sort out what is going to happen in the future. A social worker may also be involved in this type of meeting. If you have any brothers or sisters, try to get them along as well to give you moral support. Before the meeting, write down exactly what you can provide in the way of care each week and what you cannot offer. It is then up to your mother whether she then goes home with professional help to fill the gaps, or goes home with inadequate care for her needs, or opts to go into a care home. In your circumstances, it would probably be a good idea for everyone involved to actually sign a summary of what they have agreed at the meeting; it will then be a lot easier for you to stand your ground if your mother later changes her mind or denies that she has agreed to anything.

It may be possible for your mother to receive assistance under a scheme known as Direct Payments, which has been extended to include older people with care needs. In this situation, following assessment, discussion and planning with social services, she may be eligible to be given an amount of money each week which she can use to buy in the care she needs at home, rather than to receive services arranged by the local authority. Such an arrangement may give her a sense of more control and independence. However, this scheme would require her to employ and manage the individuals who provide the care, which may be more than she wishes or is able to do. Further details about this scheme should be available from your local social services office (see your telephone directory for contact details).

When a partner is in a care home

My husband is going into a nursing home. Will I be allowed to have any private time with him again?

If your husband is to have a single room, there is no reason why you should not be able to spend time alone together there during your visits. Many residents have keys to their rooms and lock the door if they wish, especially if they want to be left on their own for a time. If your husband is in a shared room, this may be a little more problematic, but it ought to be possible to arrange for some time together, perhaps in a different room. Talk to staff in the home (perhaps the manager) about this and see what they can offer to help you and your husband to maintain your relationship. Alternatively, it may be possible for you to have a short stay at the home every so often so that you can spend time together in a shared room. Again, this will need to be negotiated with the manager of the home and it is likely that there will be some charge for you to stay there.

Even though separation may be necessary, this does not mean that your relationship ends, only that it changes. In fact, many people find that their relationships actually improve, especially if they can concentrate on each other without worrying about caring responsibilities.

I can't look after my wife any more and she has been told that the only option is for her to go into a nursing home. I can't bear the thought of being separated from her. Would I be allowed to go into the home with her?

It may be possible for you to join your wife in the nursing home but there are several factors that you should consider. Do you need this type of care yourself? If not, it is unlikely that you personally would be able to obtain any help with funding, although the nursing costs for your wife should be paid by the NHS and she would have to pay for her personal care and accommodation costs. If you have plenty of savings or you own your property that is worth a great deal, you might be able to pay for both yourself and your wife. Remember, though, that this is likely to cost from about £900 each week, and such costs will increase annually. In some areas this type of care is already much more expensive than this, and you would be well advised to seek financial advice if you are thinking about this sort of commitment, which may last for quite a long time.

If you need some care, but not nursing home care (where there must be at least one trained nurse available at all times), it may be that places could be found in a dual-registered home. This is a care home with nursing facilities, and the cost may differ a little according to the extent of the help provided. Check whether you and your wife would be able to share a room, if this is what you would like, as some homes have separate areas for the two types of care provided. Assistance with funding, if necessary, might then be available from social services for both you and your wife, although it would be expected that any property you owned would be sold and the money used to pay for your care costs. (The nursing costs for your wife should be paid by the NHS.) Again, though, you need to plan for the long term and to seek advice about what might happen if you run out of money to pay towards the care and accommodation costs.

If you do not have any need for care at all, it is unlikely that you would get any help towards the cost, even for a residential home placement, for yourself.

Another important aspect to consider is that you might move

into a home and then find that the lifestyle does not suit you, and that you would rather live on your own than with a number of other people. Before finally deciding about this, it might be a good idea to have a short stay in the home, or even a number of stays over a period of time. That way you can get a fairly good idea of what it would be like to be there all the time. Going into the home for a trial period of a month or so might also have the same effect. You could then return home if you decided that communal living was not for you.

As an alternative to moving into the home with your wife, you could perhaps move to live closer to her so that you can visit as often as suits you. You could still be involved in some of her care when you visit. It might also be possible to stay at the home every so often so that you can spend time together. Even though separation is not what you would choose, many people find that, without too many caring responsibilities, their relationships improve. It might also be possible for your wife to spend brief periods at home, provided that you have enough help during these times. Discuss this with other members of the family and also with members of the stroke team at the hospital, your GP and a social worker, who can advise what sort of temporary help might be available for you at home during these periods.

14

Leisure, work and money

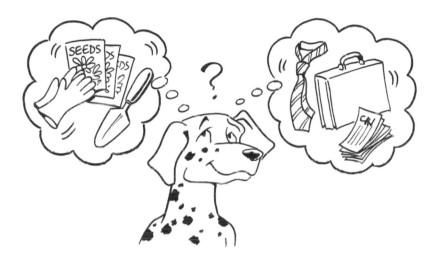

People who have been ill, including those with stroke, are often anxious to return to work. This may be because they need to earn a living or because they want to be as active as possible, or a combination of the two. People with an illness or disability that restricts the amount of work they can do may well be eligible for state benefits or possibly for grants from certain charities. Someone who spends a considerable time caring for a relative or friend may also be eligible for some help, such as Home Responsibilities Protection (which gives them credit towards state pension during time spent caring) and Carers' Allowance.

What we do in our leisure time is an important part of our lives and many people will want to return to their hobbies when they are better. Hobbies that require only gentle exercise will probably not require special consideration but it is important to ask your doctor about returning to, for example, very active sports.

Leisure

I was a keen gardener before my stroke. Will it be safe for me to carry on with this once I get over the stroke?

The more exercise you get after the stroke the better, and gardening is a very good way of keeping fit and supple. Exactly how much you will be able to do will depend on how much recovery you make. There are an increasing number of gardening implements that have been designed for people who are not as agile as they used to be – for example, long-handled trowels or shears. Electric tools can also make life much easier but don't forget to have a circuit breaker fitted to your electricity supply so that, if you accidentally cut the wire, you don't get a serious shock.

I enjoy going on long walks on the North Yorkshire moors. My family are telling me that it would be silly for me to carry on with these in case I have another stroke in the middle of nowhere. Do you think I can ignore them?

The risk of your having another stroke is not very high, especially after the first year. Our advice would be to keep doing those things that made life worth living for you and not let yourself become a prisoner of other people's fears. Do what you can to minimise the risks, though. For example, make sure you tell someone where you are going and when you expect to be back. Take a mobile phone with you if you can. As with anyone going out alone to wild parts of the country, go prepared for the worst with proper clothing, footwear and some emergency provisions. Most important of all, keep on enjoying your life.

We used to go on holiday every year to exotic places, but now that I have had a stroke I'm worried about whether I'll be able to cope with the travelling. Should we limit ourselves to holidays near our home in Scotland?

There is no doubt that travelling is a lot more stressful and tiring when your mobility is limited than for fit people. If you are dependent on a wheelchair, many parts of the world (including the UK) are not very easy places to manage in. Actually, the travelling to and from the resort will probably be fairly straightforward. If you are flying or going by train, let the carrier know in advance if you have any special needs. If you are using a travel agent, they should be able to give you advice about any particular difficulties with the journey and whether the destination you have chosen is suitable for you. Holidays are important, not least for the pleasure you get in looking forward to them. So long as you plan carefully, there should be no reason why they can't be as enjoyable as they used to be.

I want to go swimming again, but I'm frightened that, because I'm very weak down one side, I might drown.

It is possible to swim with a weak arm and leg but obviously more difficult and definitely less graceful. To begin with go with someone else who is a strong swimmer who can help you out if necessary. Better still, try to book a lesson with a swimming teacher who can give you advice on the safety of swimming and how you should adapt your technique. It may be, for example, that it would be a good idea to wear an inflated armband on the weak arm or some other sort of buoyancy aid. Swimming is a very good form of exercise after a stroke, so if it is at all possible do it!

I used to enjoy playing soccer. Is it OK for me to play again?

All strokes affect people in different ways, and everyone recovers to different levels. There certainly are people who have returned to playing football, rugby, cycling and so on. It is important, though, for each individual to ask their doctor before returning to any form of contact sport (soccer, rugby, boxing!) and to assess the risks for themselves. Non-contact sports – tennis, swimming, light exercise to music, darts – are to be encouraged as part of a general 'getting healthier' scheme. Exercise that raises your blood pressure might not be advisable in the early months of recovery after a haemorrhagic stroke but it is good for stroke survivors to be responsible for themselves and to do only what they (their bodies) feel comfortable with. Being too timid and over-cautious or being foolhardy and cavalier are to be avoided!

Are there any places where I can go to meet other young people who have had a stroke?

The Stroke Association and Different Strokes run a number of groups in the UK for younger people. Connect is an organisation that specialises in giving help and support to people with communication difficulties at least six months after stroke; they are based in London and the West of England. Contact these organisations for details (addresses in Appendix 1).

How soon can I travel by aeroplane again?

There is no absolute medical ban on flying after a stroke, but each airline has its own rules about who it allows on its planes. The oxygen pressure during flight is lower than that at sea level, so there is a theoretical risk that someone who has recently had a stroke might be harmed by flying. You should probably avoid flying for a fortnight after the stroke unless it is imperative for you to travel. After that, there is no medical reason why you shouldn't fly. Don't forget to notify the airline if you are going to need extra help at the airport or on the plane.

There is no need for you to be provided with extra oxygen on board. However, sitting in one position for a long time and becoming dehydrated can cause your blood to thicken and thus increase the risk of blood clots forming. So, if possible, get up regularly for a short walk; in any case, stretch and move your feet and legs about while you are sitting, and drink plenty of water (not alcohol!) on the flight. Remember to put your tablets (and anything else you might need on the flight) with you in your hand luggage.

Work

I want to go back to work. How can I get retrained?

First, it is important that you discuss such issues with your doctor, and perhaps with members of the specialist stroke team if one is involved. They can advise you at what point you may be recovered and well enough to return to work and what you should be aiming for. It may be, for example, that you will be able to return to your job after a sufficient period of time, depending on what that work was. It might be possible to negotiate a planned and phased return to full-time work with your employers, or to change to a part-time job if necessary. After a lengthy period of sick leave (usually more than six months), however, you are likely to need to see a health specialist. They will provide your employer with a report that contains details about your progress and whether you will be able to return to the type of work you were doing or if some alternative will be needed. If you work for a large company or a local authority, it may be possible to arrange for you to be given a different job. Your employer should then also arrange for any retraining that you might need to enable you to do this type of work.

What help is available to help me to get a job?

If you need to change jobs completely and find another employer, it will probably be useful to see a specialist at your local Employment Services JobCentre. They can also provide advice and guidance about retraining, transferable skills and rehabilitation. Many of the larger JobCentres now have specialist Disability sections (look in your telephone directory). Careers guidance about the sorts of work that might be suitable for you can be obtained through your local careers service, which may then put you in touch with the JobCentre. At the JobCentre it should be possible to see a specialist disability employment adviser (DEA) whose role is to help disabled people to find work and to facilitate access to work, particularly if there are issues relating to mobility and access. If this involves retraining, they can often help you obtain this or advise about what sorts of training to apply for. This would also be the case if you were without work before your stroke and you wanted to try to find work now. (Look in your telephone directory to find the local JobCentre and careers advice centre.) The standard of advice given by DEAs varies a bit from one area to another; if you feel that you aren't getting very much help, try voluntary groups or charities that offer such advice.

Many areas also have DIAL services (Disability Information and Advice Line) that provide advice, information and guidance for disabled people, including those who are seeking employment. The Stroke Association and Different Strokes also provide much useful advice and guidance. Some assistance may be available from charities that specialise in helping disabled people to return to work (e.g. the Shaw Trust). Some of these organisations are listed in Appendix 1.

When can I start driving again?

The Driving and Vehicle Licensing Authority (DVLA) rules that no one should drive for the first month after a stroke. Whether you can go back to driving after that depends on what problems you have been left with after the stroke and what sort of vehicle you are driving. Clearly the most important consideration must be whether you are able to drive safely, without putting you and other road users and pedestrians at risk. If, for example, you have been left with some loss of your field of vision (the area you can see when looking straight ahead), there is no possibility of being allowed to drive. If there are major problems with your perception of space and distance or memory, you won't be allowed to have your licence back. Paralysis of one side would not necessarily mean that you may not drive but you might well need to have adaptations made to your car first. Your doctor will be able to give you guidance as to whether you will be allowed to drive, but if there is any doubt you should arrange to be assessed at one of the mobility centres where you can be put through a full evaluation. They will not only tell you whether you are able to drive but also give you advice on the changes that would need to be made to your car. You must also notify your insurance company of your stroke; if you don't, they may refuse to cover you if you have an accident.

If you develop epilepsy as a result of your stroke, you must have been free of fits for a year before your licence will be returned. If you drive a public service or a heavy goods vehicle (anything over 3.5 tonnes) the regulations are much more stringent and you are likely to be refused your licence for a period of five years.

Money

What financial help might I be able to receive?

The amount of financial help available will depend to some extent on your situation before the stroke. If you had been employed for over two years, you will probably be eligible for statutory sick pay from your employer for some months following the stroke. The amount of this gradually decreases over time and a decision will be taken by a medical specialist as to whether you will be able to return to work at some point. It might be decided that you will need to retire from work on the grounds of ill health. If this is the case, you are likely to receive some form of pension and possibly also a lump-sum payment from your employer when you leave your job.

You will probably be eligible for financial assistance from the Department for Work and Pensions (DWP - formerly the Benefits Agency). There are a number of state benefits to help sick and disabled people and their dependants, and there are some payments for people who have to give up work in order to care for a sick or disabled person. These are administered by the

Disabled People and Carers unit of the DWP. By 2006, there will be integrated JobCentre Plus offices throughout the country, which will provide services to job-seekers and those people of working age in receipt of social security benefits. At present there may be separate JobCentre and social security offices in your area, so check your telephone directory for information about how to make contact with the relevant office.

You may have heard of some of the benefits that you could qualify for – Incapacity Benefit, Carer's Allowance, Attendance Allowance, Disability Living Allowance and Working Tax Credit. Some of these benefits are means-tested – your income and any savings are taken into account when they calculate the amount of assistance that you can receive. The system is fairly complex, and eligibility for such benefits varies, so it is best to obtain specialist advice; there are whole books written about such aspects, so we will not repeat them here! One in particular, the *Welfare Benefits Handbook*, is published annually by the Child Poverty Action Group (CPAG); another annual publication, intended for older people, is *Your Rights*, published by Age Concern. These books are usually available in advice centres and libraries but are also available to buy from CPAG or Age Concern. Or you could contact Disability Alliance or the Disablement Income Group, who specialise in information about benefits after an illness, or the website EntitledTo, which helps calculate your entitlement to benefits. (See Appendix 1 for contact details.)

For information and general advice about state benefits, it is probably best to contact the Benefits Enquiry Line for people with disabilities (see Appendix 1). This line can also advise you how to contact your local JobCentre Plus or social security office, where staff will be able to provide further advice and information on the various benefits, loans and grants that you might be able to obtain. (Details of your local JobCentre Plus or social security offices will also be in your local telephone directory.) The Benefits Enquiry Line has a freephone number you can ring if you need help filling in claim forms for benefits. You may also be able to get advice on your eligibility for state benefits from your social worker or the local Citizens Advice Bureau or money advice centre.

It may also be possible to obtain some financial assistance through the Independent Living (1993) Fund. This fund gives grants to help people with severe impairments, to pay for care services in their own home. To qualify, a person must be aged between 16 and 66, expect to live in the community for at least six months, be receiving the highest rate of the care component of the Disability Living Allowance and have a reduced amount of capital (e.g. savings of less than £18,500 in 2004; this excludes the value of any property but includes any capital that a partner may have). There are also conditions about the amount of services or Direct Payments that the person is receiving from social services and the need for additional services from elsewhere. The maximum money available is the combined amount from the Independent Living Fund and the social services department. Further details can be obtained from your local social services department or from the Independent Living Fund (contact details in Appendix 1).

Local branches or groups of organisations such as the Citizens Advice Bureau, Age Concern and DIAL (Disablement Information and Advice Line) are able to provide advice on financial and welfare matters. All of these organisations have information services and offer advice, information and guidance on a number of different issues. Look in the telephone directory for the ones in your area. Some national organisations such as Help the Aged (Senior Line) and Counsel and Care provide telephone helpline services; see Appendix 1 for their addresses and contact details.

Direct Payments may also be relevant for you. This cash payment scheme is generally intended to help people with needs relating to disabling conditions, and has been extended to include older people with care needs. In this situation, following assessment, discussion and planning with social services, you may be eligible to be given an amount of money each week which you then use to buy in the care you need at home rather than have the services arranged by the local authority. This can give you much greater control and independence over your circumstances although there are certain requirements. The scheme requires you to employ and manage the people who provide the care, which may be more than you either want or are able to do. Further details about this scheme should be available from your local social services office (see your telephone directory for contact details).

My husband always managed the money in our house and the bank account is in his name. He has now had a stroke and can't speak or understand what is being said to him. I need to pay the bills but the bank won't accept my signature. What can I do?

If the doctors think that it is possible that in a short time your husband will recover enough speech to be able to manage the finances again, it would be worth getting a letter from one of them to explain the situation and taking it to the bank manager. Particularly if the bills that need paying are regular out-goings, the bank will probably agree to make a special arrangement. If, however, you are likely to need to take over the money management for the long term, you will need to apply to the Court of Protection so that they can appoint someone (probably you) to manage the financial affairs. The easiest way to do this is to get a solicitor to help you. The doctor will also need to fill out a form explaining why your husband can no longer deal with the finances himself. Unfortunately, the process can take some time to organise. In the meantime your bank will make some interim arrangements.

Another possibility might have been for your husband to make a power of attorney, giving you the legal right to manage his (and your) affairs. There are two types:

- an ordinary power of attorney, which is valid only as long as the person who made it is mentally capable,

- an enduring power of attorney, which remains valid even if the person who made it becomes mentally incapable.

From what you say about your husband, though, it may not be possible for him to make a power of attorney now. Whatever the case, it would probably be wise to consult a solicitor with experience of your type of situation and seek their advice about your circumstances.

15
Research and future developments

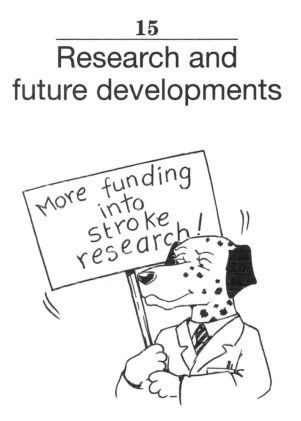

If you have read most of this book, you will be aware that there are lots of questions that get asked for which there are no definite and clear-cut answers. Much research is needed to help us understand more about stroke and to find these answers. Until recently, stroke has not attracted much funding or interest from either charities or government. This is beginning to change but stroke still gets only a tiny proportion of the research funds compared with that given to diseases such as cancer, heart disease, AIDS and diseases of children. If we are going to improve the care that is given to stroke survivors, we have to do research – and that means asking people who have had strokes to participate.

Research projects

I've been asked to take part in a research project to do with feeding after stroke. How do I know that I'm not being used as a guinea-pig?

Research on people in the UK is very carefully regulated to prevent any unethical experiments being done. All research proposals have to be submitted to a research ethics committee, which has to have on it a mixture of doctors or scientists, lay people and a lawyer. The committee must first agree that the research is worth doing. This means that the researchers must demonstrate that the question they want to answer has not already been answered satisfactorily by someone else and that the way they are proposing to do the research has a realistic chance of being successful. The committee then looks at the proposal to make sure that any people taking part in the study will not be disadvantaged in their treatment compared with others who do not participate. No research will be sanctioned if there is a significant chance of doing more harm than good.

Whoever has approached you to ask if you will take part in a research study, make sure you understand exactly what is being asked of you. Ask as many questions as you like and, if you want, get the researcher to explain it to a friend or relative as well. You should be given a written explanation of the study, written in a way that is understandable to lay people. If you want time to think about it, say so. If you do agree to take part, you will be asked to sign a consent form to show that you have had the research explained and you agree. Don't sign it just to please the doctor! Your treatment will not be adversely affected if you refuse to take part. You can withdraw from a research study at any time and without giving a reason if you so wish.

Where does the money come from to do research into stroke?

There are some stroke projects that are funded by government, through the Medical Research Council and from the European Union. The only major charity devoted to stroke research in England and Wales is The Stroke Association. In addition to the research, they also support services for people who have had stroke. The equivalent charities in Scotland and Northern Ireland are Chest, Heart & Stroke Scotland, and Northern Ireland Chest, Heart & Stroke Association. Different Strokes has also commissioned some research focusing on return to work after a stroke.

Nearly all the money these charities have has been given by the general public. Please give them your support and don't forget them when you are drawing up your will.

The future

What treatments are on the horizon that might help stroke patients?

A lot of research is being done to develop drugs that reduce the damage done at the time of a stroke. The clot-busting drug, tissue plasminogen activator (tPA), has been licensed for use in the UK but only under strict monitoring of its effects. If it is given within three hours of the first symptoms, tPA reduces the size of the stroke in some people. Other drugs being tested are aimed at reducing the damage in the brain tissue around the central stroke area, where the blood supply has not been cut off completely but has reduced blood flow and some brain function might still be saved.

There is still controversy about how intensively stroke survivors should be treated in the first few days. We don't know, for example, whether we should be controlling the blood pressure within narrow limits or monitoring and controlling the level of sugar in the blood. We hope that research will provide the answers to these questions within the next few years.

We know that people with stroke do better in stroke units where they get specialist care but what is it about those units that makes the difference, and would more of it mean that outcomes would be even better? How long should rehabilitation continue? Trying to identify exactly what the therapists do that is helpful and whether particular sorts of treatment are better than others are the subject of several research projects currently underway.

The effect of stroke on carers and the best ways of supporting them is being studied. This will, hopefully, eventually lead to better and more appropriate support for the people who do most of the work after stroke.

New drugs are being tested to try to improve stroke prevention, both for people who are at risk of stroke but have not yet had one and for people trying to prevent a recurrence. Research is underway to try to improve both the delivery of preventative treatment and people keeping up with it (compliance). At present even the proven effective treatments of controlling blood pressure and taking aspirin are not being used in all cases.

Some groups in society such as African-Caribbeans, are at particularly high risk of stroke compared with others. Whether this is due to their genes or to their environment is being investigated.

What research is going on into the recovery after stroke?

There is exciting work going on, particularly using modern technology that can give pictures not just of the structure of the brain but also of how the brain is functioning. Positron emission tomography (PET scanning) gives pictures of the brain that show where the blood is going and which bits are active. So it is possible to have someone in the scanner, give them something to read, and see the parts of the brain involved in vision, language and reading light up on the screen. This sort of technology allows researchers to monitor how the brain is recovering after a stroke, and begin to find out whether the brain is recovering by healing damaged parts or is 'switching on' bits of brain that weren't being used for that function before.

Where can I get more information about stroke and new developments in treatment?

The Stroke Association publishes a series of leaflets covering many of the aspects of stroke care, including details of the research projects it is funding. All this information is available on the website. The Association's mission is to work for a world with fewer strokes and where people touched by stroke get the help they need. Different Strokes is an organisation set up specifically to help younger people with stroke. It publishes an information pack and regular newsletters, has a website with a messageboard where stroke survivors and their carers can 'talk' to each other, and runs a nationwide network of exercise classes. It also runs workshops for child stroke survivors and their families.

The Internet has more information than anyone could possibly want. However, there is no control over what gets put onto the Internet, so you need to read with a slightly sceptical eye and not necessarily believe everything that is there. Start with reputable, recognised institutions and establishments, and see where they lead you.

Glossary

Terms in *italic* are also defined in this Glossary.

activities of daily living (ADL) The tasks that we all have to perform to lead a normal life, such as washing, dressing, using the toilet, bathing, walking and climbing stairs

agnosia The inability to recognise an object by touch alone with both hands

agraphia Difficulty writing or drawing

alexia Difficulty reading

amaurosis fugax A temporary loss of vision in one eye due to a blood clot blocking the flow of blood to the eye. There is complete recovery within 24 hours

amnesia Loss of memory

aneurysm A bulge in the wall of an artery. One of the causes of an artery leaking

angiography An X-ray or ultrasound examination of the arteries

angiomas An abnormal collection of blood vessels that can be a cause of a *haemorrhage* in the brain

angioplasty A technique whereby the doctor inserts a catheter into the narrowed portion of the artery and stretches the artery by inflating a little balloon on the end of the catheter

anticoagulant A drug that is used to 'thin' the blood and thus reduce the risk of clots forming within the circulation. The most commonly used is warfarin; another is heparin

anticonvulsants Drugs given to prevent epileptic fits

antiphospholipid syndrome A condition that results in the blood becoming stickier than normal as a result of antibodies that form against the body's phospholipids

antiplatelet therapy Drugs used to stop the *platelets* in the blood sticking to one another and forming clots. Aspirin is the most widely used. Others include clopidogrel (Plavix) and dipyridamole (Persantin)

aorta The artery taking the blood from the heart

aphasia Inability to use language. It can either be a problem understanding language (receptive) or speaking it (expressive). People are often affected by both sorts

apraxia The inability to do complex tasks when requested and there is no paralysis of the muscles

ataxia Loss of the control of muscle function, leading to a staggering walk and difficulty performing delicate tasks with the hands

atheroma The fatty deposits that build up inside an artery and eventually lead to it becoming blocked

atrial fibrillation Where the heart is beating irregularly. There is an increased risk of a blood clot forming inside the heart, which can break off, travel to the brain and cause a stroke

blood pressure Pressure needed to move the blood through the arteries

brainstem The part of the brain linking the two halves of the brain to the spinal cord. It contains some vital nerve cells to do with breathing, the heart, the eyes and many other important functions

bruit The noise that can be heard when listening over a narrowed artery

cardio-embolic stroke Stroke due to a clot that formed in the heart and travelled to the brain

carotid artery There are two carotid arteries that supply the front half of the brain with blood. Disease of a carotid artery is a common cause of stroke

carotid endarterectomy The operation that is performed to clear the inside of the *carotid artery* of *atheroma*

catheterisation The insertion of a tube inside the body. Most commonly this is into the bladder to drain the urine directly into a bag

cerebellum The part of the brain that controls fine (delicate) movement

cerebrum The largest part of the brain, made up of the left and right hemispheres (sides)

cholesterol A fatty substance that, if present in excess, can be deposited in the wall of the artery to produce *atheroma*

coma A state where someone is deeply unconscious

computed tomography (CT) The X-ray technique most commonly used to examine the brain

contractures Where a joint becomes fixed in one position by muscles that have become stiff from not being moved

deep venous thrombosis (DVT) A clot of blood in the veins, usually of the leg

delirium An temporary state of confusion, often linked with other illness such as infection

dementia A long-term (chronic) state of confusion, which can result from, for example, multiple strokes or Alzheimer's disease

disability The inability to perform normal functions, such as walking, dressing, shopping

diuretics Drugs given to make you pass more urine. They are used to control heart failure and high blood pressure

dysarthria Difficulty in speaking

dyslexia Difficulty in reading

dysphagia Difficulty in swallowing

dysphasia Difficulty in using language

dysphonia Difficulty speaking loud (or soft) enough

dyspraxia Difficulty doing complex tasks

echocardiogram An ultrasound examination of the heart

electrocardiogram (ECG) The test that records the electrical activity of the heart

embolism When a piece of solid material, usually a blood clot, travels to elsewhere in the body

emotionalism Difficulty controlling the emotions – crying and laughing easily and sometimes inappropriately

epilepsy A condition that causes fits, which can be of many different types and can occur following stroke

field of vision The area that you can see without moving your eyes (or your head)

gait The characteristics of walking

goal setting The process whereby the professionals and the patient decide on the main objectives for rehabilitation

handicap The social consequence of *disability* for the individual

haematoma A blood clot that has formed outside a blood vessel (artery or vein)

haemorrhage Where a blood vessel leaks, allowing blood to escape into the tissues – bleeding

haemorrhagic infarct An area of dead brain that has had bleeding in it

hemianopia Loss of one-half of the normal *field of vision*

hemiparesis Weakness of one-half of the body

hemiplegia Complete paralysis of half of the body

heparin An *anticoagulant* given to prevent blood clots forming

Hughes' syndrome *see* antiphospholipid syndrome

hydrocephalus Raised pressure within the skull. It can occur after a brain *haemorrhage*

hypercholesterolaemia A high level of cholesterol in the blood

hyperlipidaemia A high level of fats in the blood

hypertension High blood pressure

hypotension Low blood pressure

impairment Loss of function (e.g. weakness, loss of sensation, loss of speech)

incontinence Loss of control of passing urine or faeces

infarct/infarction An area of cell death (e.g. part of the brain) as a result of being deprived of its blood supply

intracerebral haemorrhage A *haemorrhage* inside the brain

ischaemia Cells that have an inadequate blood supply (*see also* transient ischaemic attack)

lacunar stroke A small stroke less than one centimetre in diameter

lumbar puncture A procedure whereby some of the spinal fluid is removed by the insertion of a needle into the spine

magnetic resonance angiography Using a large, powerful magnet, rather than X-rays, to create pictures of the blood vessels (arteries and veins)

magnetic resonance imaging (MRI) A type of scan that, instead of X-rays, uses a large, powerful magnet to create an image (picture) of part of the body

middle cerebral artery The artery that most frequently becomes blocked, to cause stroke

myocardial infarction The medical term for a heart attack

neglect Ignoring sensory stimuli, such as not being aware of being touched on one side or not seeing things to one side. An extreme example is not even being aware that your arm or leg belongs to you

neuroplasticity Nerve cells taking over the function of other nerve cells that are no longer functioning

nystagmus Involuntary jerking of the eyes

obesity Being more than 20% over your recommended weight

oedema Swelling

patent foramen ovale A hole in the heart that allows blood clots to get from the veins into the arteries

perception Awareness and understanding of one's environment (e.g. awareness of touch, sights, sounds)

percutaneous endoscopic gastrostomy (PEG) Insertion of a tube through the wall of the abdomen into the stomach for the purposes of feeding. It is done with a gastroscope, which is a fibre-optic instrument used to examine the inside of the stomach

platelets Small blood particles that stick together to form a clot

positron emission tomography (PET) A scanning technique that uses radioactive isotopes to show how well cells are functioning

prognosis Expected outcome

pulmonary embolism A blood clot in the lungs

rehabilitation The process of regaining function through active treatment

risk factors The possible underlying causes (for the stroke) such as smoking, high blood pressure, ethnic group, family history of stroke

spasticity The stiffness that develops in the muscles after a stroke or other type of damage to the brain or spinal cord

stenosis A narrowing

subarachnoid haemorrhage Bleeding between the brain and one of the covering membranes, often due to a leaking *aneurysm*

thalamus (thalamic) A part of the brain where the nerves carrying information about sensation from the body join with other nerves

thrombolysis The use of drugs to break up a blood clot

thrombosis The formation of a blood clot

tissue plasminogen activator (tPA) The drug most commonly used for *thrombolysis*

transient ischaemic attack (TIA) A stroke that fully recovers within 24 hours of the start of symptoms

ventricular septal defect A hole in the muscle wall that separates the two chambers (ventricles) of the heart

vertebral arteries The two arteries that travel up the back of the neck to the brain which, with the two *carotid arteries*, supply all the blood to the brain

vertigo An abnormal sensation of movement

warfarin The most frequently used oral *anticoagulant*

Appendix 1

Useful addresses

Not all the organisations listed have been mentioned in the text; they are included here in case they might be of interest. Please note that addresses, and particularly website addresses, change from time to time.

Action on Smoking and Health (ASH)
102 Clifton Street
London EC2A 4HW
Tel: 020 7739 5902
Fax: 020 7613 0531
Website: www.ash.org.uk
Information on how smoking affects medical conditions

Alzheimer's Society
Gordon House
10 Greencoat Place
London SW1P 1PH
Helpline: 0845 3000 336
   (Mon–Fri, 8 a.m.–6.30 p.m.)
Tel: 020 7306 0606
Fax: 020 7306 0808
Website: www.alzheimers.org.uk
The main charity providing information and support for people with Alzheimer's disease and their carers

Association of Charity Officers
Unicorn House
Station Close
Potters Bar
Herts EN6 3JW
Tel: 01707 651777
Fax: 01707 660477
Website: www.aco.uk.net
Advice on how to find out about charities that could help you

Afasic
2nd Floor
50–52 Great Sutton Street
London EC1V 0DJ
Helpline: 0845 355 5577
Tel: 020 7490 9410
Fax: 020 7251 2834
Website: www.afasic.org.uk
Help for people who have speech impairments

Age Concern England
1268 London Road
London SW16 4ER
Information line: 0800 00 99 66
Tel: 020 8765 7200
Fax: 020 8765 7211
Website: www.ageconcern.org.uk
*Provides advice on a range of
subjects for people over 50*

**Association of Independent
  Care Advisers**
Orchard House
Albury
Guildford GU5 9AG
Tel: 01483 203066
Fax: 01483 202535
Website: www.aica.org.uk
*Information and advice about care
options for elderly people with
learning or physical disabilities*

Benefits Enquiry Line
Tel: 0800 88 22 00
  (Mon–Fri, 8.30 a.m.–6.30 p.m.;
    Sat 9 a.m.–1 p.m.)
For help in filling in claim forms:
  0800 44 11 44
Or see the telephone directory for
  your local office
*For information on state benefits
for people with disabilities and
their carers*

British Acupuncture Council
63 Jeddo Road
London W12 9HQ
Tel: 020 8735 0400
Fax: 020 8735 0404
Website: www.acupuncture/org.uk
*Regulatory body of acupuncture
practitioners*

**British Association for
  Counselling**
BACP House
35–37 Albert Street
Rugby
Warwickshire CV21 2SG
Website: www.bacp.co.uk
*To find out about counselling
services in your area. Send s.a.e.
for information and publications
list*

British Heart Foundation
14 Fitzhardinge Street
London W1H 4DH
Helpline: 0845 070 8070
Tel: 020 7935 0185
Publications order line:
  01604 640 016
Fax: 020 7486 5820
Website: www.bhf.org.uk
*A charity funding research into
heart disease, and providing help
and advice. HeartstartUK, part
of BHF, arranges training in
emergency life-saving techniques:
tel: 020 7487 9419*

British Lung Foundation
73–75 Goswell Road
London EC1V 7ER
Tel: 020 7688 5555
Fax: 020 7688 5556
Website: www.britishlungfoundation.org
*A charity funding research into
lung disease, and providing help
and advice*

British Red Cross
9 Grosvenor Crescent
London SW1X 7EJ
Tel: 020 7235 5454
Fax: 020 7245 6315
Website: www.redcross.org.uk
*Offers quality and emergency care
to people in need, in crisis in their
own homes, community at home
and abroad. Has home aids
available for hire via its local
branches*

Calibre
New Road
Weston Turville
Aylesbury
Buckingham HP22 5XQ
Tel: 01296 432339
Fax: 01296 392599
Website: www.calibre.org.uk
*A library of over 6,000 titles for
adults and children available in
large print, on cassette, CD-ROM,
diskette and on-line for visually
impaired people.
To order the Ability Mail Order
catalogue, tel: 0116 270 1462*

Carers UK
20–25 Glasshouse Yard
London EC1A 4JT
Tel: 020 7490 8818
Fax: 020 7490 8824
Website: www.carersonline.org.uk
*Campaigns at national level on
behalf of all carers. Offers
information, advice and support
for carers. Has national
headquarters, as listed below*

Carers North of England
23 New Mount Street
Manchester M4 4DE
Tel: 0161 953 4233
Fax: 0161 953 4092
Website: www.carersonline.org.uk

Carers Northern Ireland
58 Howard Street
Belfast BT1 6PJ
Tel: 028 9043 9843
Fax: 028 9043 9299
Website: www.carersonline.org.uk

Carers Scotland
91 Mitchell Street
Glasgow G1 3LN
Tel: 0141 221 9141
Fax: 0141 221 9140
Website: www.carersonline.org.uk

Chest, Heart & Stroke Scotland
65 North Castle Street
Edinburgh EH2 3LT
Advice line: 0845 077 6000
    (Mon–Fri, 9.30 a.m.–12.30 p.m.;
    1.30–4 p.m.)
Tel: 0131 225 6963
Fax: 0131 220 6313
Website: www.chss.org.uk
*Advice and local groups for stroke
survivors in Scotland. Also funds
research into stroke*

Child Poverty Action Group
94 White Lion Street
London N1 9PF
Tel: 020 7837 7979
Website: www.cpag.org.uk
Researches and campaigns for
reform on behalf of low-income
families. Its Welfare Benefits
Handbook, *published annually,*
provides information to welfare
rights advisers. Training courses
also provided

Citizens Advice (National
   Association of Citizens
   Advice Bureaux)
Myddleton House
115–123 Pentonville Road
London N1 9LZ
Tel: 020 7833 2181
Fax: 020 7833 4371
Website: www.adviceguide.org.uk
For advice on legal, financial and
consumer matters. Good general
source of information. See your
telephone book for the one in your
area

Connect
16–18 Marshalsea Road
London SE1 1HL
Tel: 020 7367 0840
Fax: 020 7267 0841
Website: www.ukconnect.org
A national charity working with
people with communication
disability to find new ways of
'talking' and new ways of living
through an integrated programme
of therapy, education and research

Continence Foundation
307 Hatton Square
16 Baldwins Gardens
London EC1N 7RJ
Helpline: 0845 345 0165
   (Mon–Fri, 9.30 a.m.–12.30 p.m.)
Tel: 020 7404 6875
Fax: 020 7404 6876
Website:
www.continence-foundation.org.uk
For advice, and a continence
adviser near you. Also has leaflets
on incontinence

Counsel and Care
Lower Ground Floor
Twyman House
16 Bonny Street
London NW1 9PG
Helpline: 0845 300 7585
   (10.30 a.m.–1 p.m.)
Tel: 020 7241 8555
Fax: 020 7267 6877
Website: www.counselandcare.org.uk
For advice on remaining at home
or about care homes

Court of Protection
Public Guardianship Office
Archway Tower
2 Junction Road
London N19 5SZ
Helpline: 0845 330 2900
Tel: 020 7664 7000
   (Mon–Fri, 9 a.m.–5 p.m.)
Fax: 020 7664 7705
Website: www.guardianship.gov.uk
If you need to take over the
financial affairs of someone who
is mentally incapable

Crossroads – Caring for Carers
10 Regent Place
Rugby
Warwickshire CV21 2PN
Helpline: 0845 450 0350;
    Wales 029 2022 2282
Tel: 01788 573653
Fax: 01788 565498
Website: www.crossroads.org.uk
*Provides a paid, trained person to
offer respite care in the home*

**Crossroads (Scotland) Care
    Attendance Schemes**
24 George Square
Glasgow G2 1EG
Tel: 0141 226 3793
Fax: 0141 221 7130
Website:
www.crossroads.scotland.co.uk
*Provides a paid, trained person to
offer respite care in the home*

CRUSE – Bereavement Care
126 Sheen Road
Richmond
Surrey TW9 1UR
Helpline: 0870 167 1677
Bereavement Line: 0845 758 5565
Tel: 020 8940 4818
Fax: 020 8940 7638
Website:
www.crusebereavementcare.org.uk
*Offers information and practical
advice, sells literature and has
local branches that can provide
one-to-one counselling to people
who have been bereaved. Has
training in bereavement
counselling for professionals*

**Department for Work
    and Pensions**
Helpline: 0800 137 177
*Refers people with disabilities who
want to return to work and are
already on disability or
incapacity benefits, to local job
brokers who will help find
employment*

DIAL UK
St Catherine's
Tickhill Road
Doncaster DN4 8QN
Tel: 01302 310123
Fax: 01302 310404
Website: www.dialuk.org.uk
*Administrative HQ for national
network of organisations; will
refer to local centres offering
information and advice to people
with disabilities*

Different Strokes
9 Canon Harnett Court
Wolverton Mill
Milton Keynes MK12 5NF
Tel: 0845 130 71 72
Fax: 01908 313501
Website: www.differentstrokes.co.uk
*Support for younger people with
stroke*

Disability Alliance
1st Floor East
Universal house
88–94 Wentworth Street
London E1 7SA
Helpline/Minicom: 020 7247 8763
　(Mon and Wed, 2–4 p.m.)
Tel/Minicom: 020 7247 8776
　(Mon–Fri 10 a.m.–4 p.m.,
　publications only)
Fax: 020 7247 8765
Website: www.disabilityalliance.org
*Campaigns for a better deal for
people with disabilities. Publishes*
Disability Rights Handbook,
*regularly up-dated, giving
information on disability welfare
benefits*

Disability Information Trust
Mary Marlborough Centre
Nuffield Orthopaedic Centre
Headington
Oxford OX3 7LD
Tel: 01865 227592
Fax: 01865 227596
Website:
www.home.btconnect.com/trust/home.htm
*Assesses/tests disability
equipment on the market and
publishes findings*

Disability Law Service
39–45 Cavell Street
London E1 2BP
Tel: 020 7791 9800
Textphone: 020 7791 9801
Fax: 020 7791 9802
Website: www.dls.org.uk
*Free legal advice for disabled
people and their carers and
families*

Disabled Drivers Association
National HQ
Ashwellthorpe
Norwich
Norfolk NR16 1EX
Tel: 0870 770 3333
Fax: 01508 488173
Website: www.dda.org.uk
*Information and advice for
disabled drivers*

Disabled Drivers' Motor Club
Cottingham Way
Thrapston
Northants NN14 4PL
Tel: 01832 734724
Fax: 01832 733816
Website: www.ddmc.org.uk
*Information and advice about
mobility problems for disabled
people*

**Disabled Living Centres
　Council**
Redbank House
4 St Chad's Street
Manchester M8 8QA
Helpline: 0870 770 2866
Tel: 0161 834 1044
Textphone: 0161 839 0885
Fax: 0161 839 2867
Website: www.dlcc.org.uk
*Co-ordinates the work of Disabled
Living Centres UK-wide, which
have information and advice
about products that can increase
disabled or older people's choices
about how they live. Offers
training courses for professionals*

Disabled Living Foundation
380–384 Harrow Road
London W9 2HU
Tel: 020 7289 6111
Helpline: 0845 130 9177
   (Mon–Fri, 10 a.m.–1 p.m.)
Fax: 020 7266 2922
Textphone: 020 7432 8009
Website: www.dlf.org.uk
*For information about equipment
to help you cope with a disability*

**Disablement Income Group
   (DIG) Scotland**
5 Quayside Street
Edinburgh EH6 6EJ
Tel: 0131 555 2811
Fax: 0131 554 7076
Website: www.digscotland.org.uk
*Provides welfare benefits
information and advice service to
disabled people and their carers
throughout Scotland*

**Elderly Accommodation
   Counsel**
3rd Floor
89 Albert Embankment
London SE1 7TP
Tel: 020 7820 1343
Fax: 020 7820 3970
Website: www.housingcare.org.uk
*Information about all forms of
accommodation for older people*

EntitledTo
Website: www.entitledto.co.uk
*Helps you work out your
entitlement to state benefits and
tax credits*

**Greater London Association
   for Disabled People (GLAD)**
336 Brixton Road
London SW9 7AA
Tel: 020 7346 5800
Fax: 020 7346 5810
Website: www.glad.org.uk
*Information for disabled people in
the London area*

**Headway (The Brain Injury
   Association)**
4 King Edward Court
King Edward Street
Nottingham NG1 1EW
Helpline: 0808 800 2244
Tel: 0115 924 0800
Textphone: 0115 950 7825
Fax: 0115 958 4446
Website: www.headway.org.uk
*For people who are disabled
physically or mentally as a result
of a head injury, and their carers*

Health Information Service
Tel: 0800 66 55 44 (10 a.m.–4 p.m.)
*Information leaflets on healthy
eating, keeping fit and weight
reduction*

Help the Aged
207–221 Pentonville Road
London N1 9UZ
Helpline: 0808 800 6565;
   N Ireland 0808 808 7575
Tel: 020 7278 1114
Fax: 020 7278 1116
Website: www.helptheaged.org.uk
*Advice and support for older
people and carers*

Holiday Care
7th Floor, Sunley House
4 Bedford Park
Croydon CR0 2AP
Helpline: 0845 124 9971
Tel: 0845 124 9974
Fax: 0845 124 9972
Website: www.holidaycare.org.uk
*Information and advice about
holidays, travel or respite care for
older or disabled people and carers*

**Independent Living (1993)
  Fund**
PO Box 7525
Nottingham NG2 4ZT
Helpline: 0845 601 8815
Fax: 0115 945 0948
Website: www.ilf.org.uk
*May fund very severely disabled
people to buy in extra care*

INTACT
Speech and Language Therapy
Research Unit
North Bristol NHS Trust
Frenchay Hospital
Bristol BS16 1LE
Tel: 0117 918 6529
Fax: 0117 970 1119
Website: www.speech-therapy.org.uk
*INTACT is a computer program
for speech*

Jewish Care
Stuart Young House
221 Golders Green Road
London NW11 9DQ
Helpline: 020 8922 2222
(Emergency out-of-hours:
  0800 413 285)
Tel: 020 8922 2000
Fax: 020 8922 1998
Website: www.jewishcare.org
*Social care, personal support and
residential homes for Jewish
people*

John Groom's
45/50 Scrutton Street
London EC2A 4XQ
Tel: 020 7452 2000
Fax: 020 7452 2001
Website: www.johngrooms.org.uk
*Helps people with disabilities to
live as independently as possible
and offers residential, respite and
holiday accommodation*

**Kings Healthcare Rehabilitation
  Centre**
Assistive Technology Team
Bowley Close
Farquhar Road
London SE19 1SZ
Tel: 020 7346 5220
Fax: 020 7346 5234
*For information about assessment
of assistive technology (prostheses,
orthotics and wheelchairs) to
people in Southwark, Lewisham
and Lambeth*

Leonard Cheshire
30 Millbank
London SW1P 4QD
Tel: 020 7802 8200
Fax: 020 7802 8250
Website: www.leonard-cheshire.org
Provides a range of help,
including residential homes and
home care attendants for disabled
people

London Mobility Unit
New Zealand House
80 Haymarket
London SW1Y 4TZ
Tel: 020 7484 2929
Fax: 020 7839 7478
Advice about concessionary fares
(Freedom Pass) and Taxicards in
the London area

Mobility Advice and Vehicle
    Information Service (MAVIS)
Department of Transport
Crowthorne Business Estate
Old Wokingham Road
Crowthorne
Berkshire RG45 6XD
Tel: 01344 661000
Fax: 01344 661066
Website: www.mobility-unit.dft.gov.uk
Advice on car adaptations and
transport for disabled people

Motability
Goodman House
Station Approach
Harlow
Essex CM20 2ET
Helpline: 0845 456 4566
Tel: 01279 635999
Textphone: 01279 632273
Fax: 01279 632000
Website: www.motability.co.uk
Advice and help about cars,
scooters and wheelchairs for
disabled people

Naidex
Touchstone Exhibitions &
    Conferences Ltd
Haleon House
4 Red Lion Street
Richmond
Surrey TW9 1RW
Tel: 020 8332 0044
Fax: 020 8332 0874
Website: www.t-stone.co.uk
Holds exhibitions of aids and
equipment to help disabled people

National Association of
    Councils for Voluntary
    Service
3rd Floor, Arundel Court
177 Arundel Street
Sheffield S1 2NU
Tel: 0114 278 6636
Textphone: 0114 278 7025
Fax: 0114 278 7004
Website: www.nacvs.org.uk
Promotes and supports the work of
Councils for Voluntary Service by
working with groups in the
community

**National Association of Funeral
Directors**
618 Warwick Road
Solihull
Birmingham B91 1AA
Helpline: 0845 230 1343
Tel: 0121 711 1343
Fax: 0121 711 1351
Website: www.nafd.org.uk
*Trade association of funeral
directors offering a code of
conduct for a simple funeral*

**National Council for Voluntary
Organisations (NCVO)**
Regents Wharf
8 All Saints Street
London N1 9RL
Tel: 020 7713 6161
Fax: 020 7713 6300
Website: www.ncvo-vol.org.uk
*Information on local voluntary
organisations that may be able to
provide help*

NHS Direct
England and Wales: 0800 66 55 44
*Speak to a nurse for some
common-sense advice about your
health*

NHS 24
Scotland: 0800 22 44 88
*Speak to a nurse for some
common-sense advice about your
health*

NHS Smoking Helpline
Helpline: 0800 169 0 169
*NHS helpline for help and advice
on giving up smoking*

**Northern Ireland Chest, Heart
& Stroke Association**
22 Great Victoria Street
Belfast BT2 7LX
Helpline: 08457 697 298
Tel: 028 9032 0184
Fax: 028 9033 3487
Website: www.nichsa.com
*Advice and support for stroke
survivors in Northern Ireland*

Outsiders Club
Sex and Disability Helpline
Tuppy Owens
BCM Box Lovely
London WC1N 3XX
Tel: 0707 499 3527 (11 a.m.–7 p.m.)
Website: www.outsiders.org.uk
*A national self-help organisation
that helps with sexual problems*

Pensions Advisory Service
11 Belgrave Road
London SW1V 1RB
Helpline: 0845 601 2923
Fax: 020 7233 8016
Website: www.opas.org.uk
*A voluntary organisation that
helps with queries and problems to
do with occupational and personal
pensions*

Phab
Summit House
Wandle Road
Croydon
Surrey CR0 1DF
Tel: 020 8667 9443
Fax: 020 8681 1399
Website: www.phabengland.org.uk
*Works to promote integration
between disabled and non-disabled
people on equal terms*

Princess Royal Trust for Carers
142 Minories
London EC3N 1LB
Tel: 020 7480 7788
Fax: 020 7481 4729
Website: www.carers.org
Provides information on a UK-wide network of independent carer centres as well as support and practical help for carers; your phone book may list a local branch

Glasgow Office
Campbell House
215 West Campbell Street
Glasgow G2 4TT
Tel: 0141 221 5066
Fax: 0141 221 4623
Website: www.carers.org

Northern Office
Suite 4, Oak House
High Street
Chorley PR7 1DW
Tel: 01257 234070
Fax: 01257 234105
Website: www.carers.org

Quit
Ground Floor
211 Old Street
London EC1V 9NR
Helpline: 0800 00 22 00
(Scotland 0800 84 84 84)
Tel: 020 7251 1551
Fax: 020 7251 1661
Website: www.quit.org.uk
Charity offering individual advice on giving up smoking, in English and Asian languages. Talks to schools on smoking and pregnancy and can refer to local groups

RADAR (Royal Association for Disability and Rehabilitation
12 City Forum
250 City Road
London EC1V 8AF
Tel: 020 7250 3222
Fax: 020 7250 0212
Website: www.radar.org.uk
Campaigns to improve the rights and care of disabled people. Sells special key to access locked public toilets for the disabled

REACT
Propeller Multimedia Ltd
PO Box 13791
Peebles EII45 9YR
Tel/Fax: 01896 833528
Website: www.propeller.net/rehab
REACT is a computer program for speech

Registered Nursing Homes Association
15 Highfield Road
Edgbaston
Birmingham B15 3DU
Helpline: 0800 0740 194
Tel: 0121 454 2511
Fax: 0121 454 0932
Website: www.rnha.co.uk
Information about registered nursing homes in your area that meet the standards set by the Association

Relate (formerly **National Marriage Guidance Council**)
Herbert Gray College
Little Church Street
Rugby
Warwickshire CV21 3AP
Helpline: 0845 130 4010
  for counselling
Tel: 01788 573241 or 0845 456 1310
  for general information
Fax: 01788 535007
Website: www.relate.org.uk
Offers relationship counselling via local branches. Relate publications on health, sexual, self-esteem, depression, bereavement and remarriage issues available from bookshops, libraries or via website

Relatives and Residents Association
24 The Ivories
6–18 Northampton Street
London N1 2HY
Helpline: 020 7359 8136
Tel: 020 7359 8148
Fax: 020 7226 6603
Website: www.relres.org.uk
Support and advice for older relatives and friends of people in care homes or hospital long-term

Remploy Ltd
Stonecourt
Siskin Drive
Coventry CV3 4FJ
Tel: 024765 15800
Website: www.remploy.co.uk
Has 96 factories around the UK, employing people with disabilities in a variety of manufacturing fields. Gives advice about returning to work

Scottish Association for Mental Health
Cumbrae House
15 Carlton Court
Glasgow G5 9JP
Tel: 0141 568 7000
Fax: 0141 568 7001
Website: www.samh.org.uk
Information about services in Scotland for people with mental health problems

Scottish Council for Voluntary Organisations
The Mansfield
Traquair Centre
15 Mansfield Place
Edinburgh EH3 6BB
Tel: 0131 556 3882
Textphone: 0131 557 6483
Fax: 0131 556 0279
Website: www.scvo.org.uk
For information about voluntary organisations in Scotland

Sexual Dysfunction Association
Windmill Place Business Centre
2–4 Windmill Lane
Southall UB2 4NU
Helpline: 0870 774 3571
Website: www.sda.uk.net
Help and advice on sexual problems

Shaftesbury Housing Group
16 Kingston Road
London SW19 1JZ
Tel: 020 8239 5555
Fax: 020 8239 5580
Website: www.shaftesburysoc.org.uk
*Christian society providing
residential centres, schools,
colleges and holiday centres for
disabled people of all religious
faiths. Has prayer line*

Shaw Trust
Shaw House, Epsom Square
White Horse Business Park
Trowbridge
Wilts BA14 0XJ
Tel: 01225 716350
Fax: 01225 716334
Minicom: 08457 697 288
Website: www.shaw-trust.org.uk
*Advice to help people with
disabilities return to work*

**Soldiers, Sailors, Airmen
and Families Association
(SSAFA Forces Help)**
19 Queen Elizabeth Street
London SE1 2LP
Tel: 020 7403 8783
Fax: 020 7403 8815
Website: www.ssafa.org.uk
*National charity offering
information, advice and financial
aid to serving and ex-service men
and women and their families
who are in need*

Speakability (formerly **Action
for Dysphasic Adults**)
1 Royal Street
London SE1 7LL
Helpline: 0808 808 957
Tel: 020 7261 9572
Fax: 020 7928 9542
Website: www.speakability.org.uk
*Help for adults with language
problems (aphasia). Has
literature and local support groups*

Stroke Association
Stroke House
240 City Road
London EC1V 2PR
Helpline: 0845 30 33 100
Fax: 020 7490 2686
Website: www.stroke.org.uk
*National charity providing
comprehensive information and
advice about stroke illness, with
community services around the
country. Major funder of stroke
research*

Tripscope
Vassal Centre
Gill Avenue
Bristol BS16 2QQ
Helpline: 08457 585 641
Fax: 0117 939 7736
Website: www.tripscope.org.uk
*Information and advice about
travel and transport for disabled
and older people and their carers
in the UK and abroad*

UK Home Care Association (UKHCA)
42B Banstead Road
Carshalton Beeches
Surrey SM5 3NW
Tel: 020 8288 1551
Fax: 020 8288 1550
Website: www.ukhca.co.uk
Offers information about member organisations with a code of practice providing home care in your area

Ulster Cancer Foundation
Pavilion 2
Belvoir Park Hospital
Hospital Road
Belfast BT8 8JR
Tel: 028 9049 2007
Fax: 028 9069 3376
Website: www.ulstercancer.org
Offers a helpline for people wanting to give up smoking.

Wales Council for Voluntary Action
Baltic House
Mount Stuart Square
Cardiff CF10 5FH
Helpline: 0870 607 1666
Fax: 029 2043 1701
Website: www.wcva.org.uk
Information about voluntary groups in Wales

Women's Royal Voluntary Service (WRVS)
Garden House
Milton Hill
Abingdon
Oxon OX13 6AD
Tel: 01235 442900
Fax: 01235 861166
Website: www.wrvs.org.uk
Provides a range of services in the community; often provides meals-on-wheels

Appendix 2

Useful publications

Care after Stroke: Information for patients and their carers by Marcia Kelson and Penny Irwin (based on the NHS Executive's *National Clinical Guidelines for Stroke*), published by the Royal College of Physicians, London (2000)

Caring for Someone who has had a Stroke by Philip Coyne with Penny Mares, published by Age Concern England, London (1995)

A Guide to Grants for Individuals in Need edited by S Harland, published by the Directory of Social Change, London (1998/9)

My Year Off by Robert McCrum, published by Picador, London (1998)

Index

Note Page numbers in *italics* refer to diagrams or tables. Page numbers followed by italic *g* indicate Glossary entries.

abscess of brain *19*
accommodation *see* care home; family as carers; home care; sheltered housing
ACE (angiotensin-converting enzyme) inhibitors 164
activities of daily living (ADL) 139, 227*g*
    see also aids and equipment
acupuncture 67, 124
Adalat (nifedipine) 126
ADL *see* activities of daily living
Afro-Caribbean people 157, 165, 224
age
    diet after stroke 79
    and stroke incidence 43–4
    young people 49–50, 160–2, 191, 214
Age Concern 218, 219
agnosia 227*g*

agraphia 93–4, 227*g*
aids and equipment 61–4, 74
    for communication 94–5
    cost 142–3
    daily living 139–40, 142–4
    on discharge from hospital 179–80
    from Red Cross 65, 143
    urinary incontinence 98–9
    see also walking; wheelchairs
airway (trachea) 69
alcohol *19*
alexia 134, 227*g*
Aloprostadil 198
Alzheimer's disease 109
amaurosis fugax 8, 227*g*
amitriptyline 114, 123
amlodipine 164–5
amnesia 227*g*
    see also memory loss
amphetamines 163
anaemia 163
aneurysm 9–10, 27, 36, 162, 227*g*
    affecting childbirth 201
    urgent repair 174
angio-oedema 167
angiography 24, 227*g*, 230*g*

angioma 227*g*
angioplasty, carotid 173–4
angiotensin-converting enzyme
    (ACE) inhibitors 164
anticoagulants 29–30, 158, 169,
    223, 227*g*
anticonvulsants 123, 227*g*
antidepressants 114, 117, 123–4
antioxidants 84–5
antiphospholipid syndrome
    163, 201, 227*g*
antiplatelet therapy 227–8*g*
anus 102
anxiety 110
aorta 4, 7, 172, 228*g*
aortic stenosis 157
aphasia 115, 228*g*
apnoea during sleep 159–60
apraxia 228*g*
aromatherapy 67, 128
arteries 4–6, *6*, *7*, 8, 12
    carotid 5, 26, 155, 172,
        172–3, 228*g*
    cerebral *6*, *7*
    dissection of artery 162
    effect of stress 153
    high blood pressure 148
    infective endocarditis 163
    middle cerebral artery *6*,
        230*g*
    problems and risk 162
    recovery after stroke 13–14
    value of antioxidants 84–5
    vasculitis 162
    vertebral 5, *6*, 12, 163, 232*g*
    see also cholesterol;
        haemorrhage; infarct/
        infarction

arterio-venous malformation
    (AVM) 10–11, *19*, 162
arteriogram 27, 172
arthritis 126
Asasantin (dipyridamole) 168
    see also Persantin
aspiration (food in airway) 69
aspirin 8, 24, 31, 158, 159
    allergy to 168
    alternatives 168
    and brain scan 33
    dosage 167
    importance and function
        165–6
    side effects 34, 167, 170
    see also warfarin
asthma 165
ataxia 228*g*
atenolol 165
atheroma 12, *12*, 26, 148, 157,
    228*g*
atrial fibrillation 12, 158–9,
    169, 170, 228*g*
AVM *see* arterio-venous
    malformation

baclofen 58, 128
balance 17, 39, 136–7
ball, exercise 64
ballooning of artery *see*
    aneurysm
barium swallow 29
bed-wetting *see* incontinence
bedpans 99
beds and safety 45–6
bendrofluazide 164
benefits (state) 217–18
betahistine (Serc) 137

bladder *see* incontinence; urinary problems
bleeding 167, 170
see also haemorrhage
blockage *see* infarct/infarction
blood
  cells 7, 13
  chemistry abnormalities *19*
  clotting *see* clotting of blood problems and risk 163
  supply to brain 4–6, *6, 7*
  tests 27, 169
  see also haemorrhage
blood pressure
  Afro-Caribbean people 165
  high (hypertension) 9, 35, 79–80, 200, 228*g*
  as risk factor 148–50, 156
  normal 149–50
  problems and risk 163
  reducing 150
blood sugar 160
BMI *see* Body Mass Index
Bobath Cuff support 55
Body Mass Index (BMI) 82–4, *83*
botulinum toxin 58–9
bowels *see* constipation; incontinence, bowels
brain
  cells 13–14
  extent of damage 16, 20–2
  function 3–6, *4–6*
  recovery after stroke 13–14
  stroke-like symptoms 18, *19*
  see also headache, possible causes

brain scan 24–5, 126, 155, 176
  see also computed tomography (CT) scan; magnetic resonance imaging (MRI)
brainstem 3, *5*, 68, 137, 228*g*
breathing problems 21
bruit (sound) 26, 228*g*
butter 77, 78

capillaries 10–11
captopril 164
carbamazepine (Tegretol) 123, 176
cardiac catheterisation 157–8
cardio-embolic stroke 228*g*
cardiologist 156, 157
care *see* care home; intensive care; respite care; sheltered housing; social services
care home 181–2, 183–4, 187–92
  accompanied by partner 208–9
  choosing one 188–90
  for disabled people 191
  for younger people 191
  nursing home 190–1
carers
  Carer Assessment 179
  day care 204
  protecting own health 206–7
  relatives as carers 182–3, 184–6, 202–8
  research on support 224
  'sitting service' for respite 186
  support groups 204–5

Carers' Allowance 211
carotid angioplasty 173–4
carotid endarterectomy 26, 172–3
carotid ultrasound (doppler) 26
catheter
    cardiac 157–8
    urinary 98–9, 196–7, 228*g*
cerebellum 3, *4, 5,* 35, 89, 137, 228*g*
cerebro-vascular accident (CVA) 10
cerebrum 10, 228*g*
    see also hemispheres of brain
cheese 78
Child Poverty Action Group 218
chlorpromazine 176
cholesterol 7, 76–9, 229*g*
    family history 79
    fats in diet 77–8, 171
    ideal level 78, 171
    see also atheroma
cimetidine 34
circle of Willis 5–6, *6*
Citizens Advice Bureau 184, 219
clinical trials 29–30
    aspirin 33
    aspirin with dipyridamole 168
clopidogrel (Plavix) 34, 168, 169
clotting of blood 7–8, 10, 12–13, 32, 35–6
    abnormalities of mechanism 163

in heart chambers 157–8
subdural haematoma 18
    see also aspirin; drugs, clot-busting; thrombolysis; thrombosis
co-danthramer 103
cocaine 162
codeine 102
collagen 162
coma 17, 229*g*
communication aids 94–5
Community Care Assessment 179–80
complementary therapies 36–7, 67, 150
comprehension *see* understanding
computed tomography (CT) scan 16–17, 23–4, 25, 229*g*
computers as aids 94–5
concentration 111
confusion 58, 109, 114, 181–2
constipation 34, 102–4
consultants *see* specialists (medical)
contraception (the Pill) 160, 202
contractures 59, 229*g*
convalescence 183–4
cooling technique 35
cost of care *see* finance
cot sides for hospital beds 45
counselling 144–5, 182, 206–7
cramp in legs 128
cranberry juice 102
CT *see* computed tomography (CT) scan
cushions, special 106, 107

CVA (cerebro-vascular accident) 10

dantrolene 58
DDAVP (desmopressin) 101
deafness 136–7
death 19–22
deep venous thrombosis 229g
delirium 229g
dementia 109, 170
Department for Work and Pensions (DWP) 217–18
depression 109, 110, 112–16, 119
  see also electro-convulsive therapy (ECT)
desmopressin (DDAVP) 101
diabetes 18, 160, 164
diagnosis 18
DIAL see Disability Information and Advice Line
diarrhoea 102
diazepam (Valium) 128
diclofenac (Voltarol) 125
diet see food and drink
dietitian 74, 75
Different Strokes 216, 225
diplopia (double vision) 135–6
dipyridamole (Persantin) 34, 126, 168
Direct Payments scheme 180, 192, 207–8, 219
Disability Information and Advice Line (DIAL) 216, 219
Disability Living Allowance 192, 219
Disabled Living Centres 65

dislocation of joint 55
'disowning' parts of own body 117–18
dissection of artery 162
diuretics 164, 229g
dizziness 137
doctor
  GP 193–4, 205
  hospital 37
doppler see carotid doppler
doppler probe 27–8
doxazosin 165
drinks and swallowing difficulties 70
drip, fluid 32, 70, 71
driving 216–17
drowsiness 17–18, 58, 114, 123
drugs
  ACE inhibitors 164
  alpha-blockers 165
  anticoagulants 29–30, 158, 169, 223, 227g
  anticonvulsants 123, 227g
  antidepressants 114, 117, 123–4
  anti-epileptics 175–6
  beta-blockers 165
  bought over counter 127
  calcium antagonists 164–5
  clot-busting 29–30, 223, 227g
  controlling incontinence 101, 102–3
  diuretics 164, 229g
  need to persevere 114–15
  neuroprotectors 31
  non-NHS 37
  pain-killers 59, 107, 124
  reducing muscle stiffness 58

drugs (*continued*)
  research and development
    223–4
  sleeping tablets 119–21
  SSRIs 114
  statins 77, 79, 171
  steroids 60–1
  stimulant-like 163
  stroke prevention 164–71
  thiazide diuretics 164
  *see also individual drug
    names*
DVT (deep venous
    thrombosis) 229*g*
dysarthria 89, 94, 229*g*
dysgraphia 93, 94
dyslexia 93, 229*g*
dysphasia, expressive/
    receptive 86–8, 94, 229*g*
dyspraxia 229*g*

ECG *see* electrocardiogram
echocardiogram 155, 229*g*
  trans-oesophageal 27–8
ecstasy (drug) 163
ECT *see* electro-convulsive
    therapy
EEG *see* electro-
    encephalogram
eggs 77
electro-convulsive therapy
    (ECT) 115
electrocardiogram (ECG) 155,
    229*g*
electroencephalogram (EEG)
    176
electromyography 58–9
embolism 12, 20, 229*g*, 231*g*

emergencies 30
  TIA 8–9
  warning signs of stroke
    174–5
emotionalism/emotional
    lability 116, 144–5, 195,
    229*g*
employment *see* work
enalapril 164
endarterectomy, carotid 26,
    228*g*
endoscopy 71
enemas 102, 103–4
enzymes 164
Epanutin (phenytoin) 176
epilepsy 11, *19*, 175, 217, 229*g*
Epilim (sodium valproate)
    176
equipment and aids *see* aids
    and equipment
ethical considerations 19–22,
    72
exercise 76, 81–2, 119, 150
  see also occupational
    therapy; physiotherapy
extrasystoles 158
eyes/eyesight *see* vision

face
  facial expression 113, 115
  tingling sensation 129
faeces *see* incontinence,
    bowels
falling down 45–6
family as carers 182–3, 184–6,
    202–8
family history *see* heredity
family planning 201–2

fatigue 60, 63, 118–19
fats in diet *see* cholesterol
FEES *see* fibreoptic
    endoscopic evaluation of
    swallowing
ferrules on walking sticks 62
FES (functional electrical
    stimulation) 60
fibreoptic endoscopic
    evaluation of swallowing
    (FEES) 29
finance and help 180, 184,
    188–92, 205, 209, 217–20
  inability to manage finance
    220
fish 78
fitness centres 60, 62
Flowtron machine 129
fluid intake 32, 39
fluoxetine (Prozac) 114, 116
flying 214–15
food and drink
  appetite loss 73–4
  care with cooking 77
  diet for weight loss 80–4
  drinking water 73
  helpful equipment 139
  keeping food diary 80–1
  nutrition and diet 75–85
    see also weight
  puréed 70
  swallowing problems 68–75
  taste and smell problems
    136
  tube feeding 70–2, 74–5
    see also cholesterol
football 213–14
forgetfulness *see* memory loss

free radicals 84–5
frontal lobe 4, *4*
'frozen shoulder' 55, 125
functional electrical
    stimulation (FES) 60

gabapentin 124
gait *see* walking
gardening 212
gastroscopy 29, 71, 72
gastrostomy 71, 72, 231*g*
glyceryl trinitrate (GTN) 126
goal-setting 229*g*
gout 164
GP (general practitioner)
    193–4, 205
GTN (glyceryl trinitrate) 126
gymnasium *see* fitness centres

haematoma 230*g*
  subdural 18, *19*
haemorrhage 167, 170
  cerebral 8, 9, 13, 24, 230*g*
  intracerebral 8, 196, 230*g*
  subarachnoid 8, 9–10, 27, 28,
    231*g*
    from aneurysm 201
    treatment 36
hallucinations 117
hand problems 58–9, 128–9,
    139
handicap 230*g*
head injury *19*
headache
  after lumbar puncture 28
  possible causes 126, 165
  severe 9–10
hearing and balance 136–7

heart 7, 12, 27–8
heart conditions
    aortic stenosis 157
    aspirin treatment 166
    atrial fibrillation 12, 158–9,
        169, 170, 228*g*
    irregular beats 124, 158, 169
    mitral stenosis 157
    murmurs 156–7
    patent foramen ovale (hole)
        163, 231*g*
    and stroke 76, 157–9, 163
    ventricular septal defect
        157, 232*g*
Heart Protection Study 171
Help the Aged 219
help at home *see* home care
hemi-neglect 130–1, 231*g*
hemianopia 133, 135, 230*g*
hemiparesis 230*g*
hemiplegia 230*g*
hemispheres of brain 3–5, *5*,
        90–1
heparin 32, 230*g*
heredity 147–8
hiccups after strokes 176
hip pain 127–8
hobbies 154, 212, 214
hoist for lifting 44–5
holidays 180, 213
home care 39–40, 41–2, 49,
        177–84
    adaptations to property
        142–3
    occupational therapy 140–2
    relative as carer 182–3
    voluntary organisations 180
    see also hospital care

Home Responsibilities
        Protection 211
homoeopathy 150
hormone replacement therapy
        (HRT) 161, 172
hospital care 33
    complaints 194
    discharge 177, 193
    outpatients department 193
    stroke units 40–1, 43–4,
        49–50
    variety of staff 37–8, 41
    ward vs single room 46–7, 48
    see also care home;
        convalescence; home
        care; nursing home
HRT *see* hormone replacement
        therapy
Hughes' syndrome 163, 201,
        230*g*
humerus 55, 125
hydrocephalus 35, 230*g*
hydrotherapy 62–3
hygiene 96
hypercholesterolaemia 230*g*
    see also cholesterol
hyperlipidaemia 230*g*
    see also cholesterol, fats in
        diet
hypertension 230*g*
    see also blood pressure,
        high
hypotension 230*g*

ibuprofen (Nurofen) 125, 127
imipramine 114
immune system problems 163
impotence 197–8

incontinence 96–103, 230*g*
  aids 98–9
  bowels 97, 102–3
  drugs 101
  training the bladder 100
  urine 97–102
  see also pressure sores; skin
    care
Independent Living (1993)
    Fund 192, 219
infarct/infarction 9, 10, 24, 196,
    230*g*
  haemorrhagic 230*g*
  myocardial 231*g*
  treated with aspirin 31, 166
infection 57, 71, 72, 75
  inner ear 137
  skin 104–5
  urinary 100, 101–2
infective endocarditis 163
information on stroke 42
insulin 160
INTACT computer program 95
intensive care 33
investigations 23–9
ischaemic stroke 33, 230*g*
isosorbide mononitrate 126

JobCentres 215–16

knee pain 127–8

lactulose 103
language *see* speech problems
laxatives 102, 103
LDLs (low-density
    lipoproteins) 76
leg stiffness 59

leisure 211–15
ligaments 125
lipid clinic 79
lisinopril 164
living wills 21–2
lofepramine 114
loperamide 102
losartan 164
low-density lipoproteins 76
lumbar puncture 28, 230*g*

magnetic resonance
    angiography 24, 230*g*
magnetic resonance imaging
    (MRI) 23–4, 25, 230*g*
maprotiline 23, 114
massage 67, 124, 128
mattresses, special 31, 106, 107
meat 77
meditation 154
memory loss (amnesia)
    109–12, 154, 227*g*
menopause 161
metoprolol 165
mexilitene 124
'midline' awareness 52
migraine 18, 126
milk and milk products 77
mineral supplements 74
mini-stroke 9
mitral stenosis 157
money *see* finance
mood disturbance 110, 112–18
morphine 124
mouth problems 69, 114, 123
Movicol 103
MRI *see* magnetic resonance
    imaging

muscle stiffness/weakness 10,
    57–61
    see also cramp in legs;
        drugs, reducing muscle
        stiffness; dysarthria;
        dyspraxia; functional
        electrical stimulation;
        hand problems; leg
        stiffness; neck; physio-
        therapy, therapist's role
        and training; shoulder
        problems
music and speech 90
myocardial infarction 231g

nasogastric tube 70, 71, 72
neck 10, 162
neglect 130–1, 135, 231g
neuroplasticity 14, 231g
nifedipine (Adalat) 126, 164
'nil by mouth' care 69–70, 73
nimodipine 36
non-invasive positive-pressure
        ventilation (NIPPV) 160
nortriptyline 114
nose see nasogastric tube
numbness 175, 200
Nurofen (ibuprofen) 125, 127
nurses
    care at home 180
    hospital 37, 44–6
    specialist continence
        advisers 97–8, 99–100
nursing home 190–1
    see also care home
nystagmus 231g

obesity 231g

occupational therapy 37, 66,
    74, 138–43
    home care 179
    and physiotherapy 141
oedema 167, 231g
    see also swelling
oesophagus 27–8, 69
oestrogen 160
oral hygiene see mouth
        problems; teeth care
osteoarthritis 127
osteoporosis 161
outcome see prognosis
overweight 75–6, 80–3, 84, 150
oxybutynin 101
oxygen
    in blood 8, 12–13, 32–3, 35
    during sleep 159–60

pain 20–1, 113, 122–9
    central post-stroke pain
        123–4
pain clinics 124
palpitation 158
paracetamol 107, 125, 126, 127
paralysis 10, 17, 36, 39
    hemiplegia 230g
parietal lobe 4, 4, 117
paroxetine 114
patent foramen ovale 163, 231g
PEG see percutaneous
        endoscopic gastrostomy
penis 198
pensions 217
perception 117–18, 231g
percutaneous endoscopic
        gastrostomy (PEG) 71,
        231g

see also gastrostomy
perindopril 164
Persantin (dipyridamole) 34,
   126, 168
perseveration 90–1
personal care 96
personality change 108,
   113–14
PET *see* positron emission
   tomography
phenytoin (Epanutin) 176
photophobia 10
physiotherapy 14, 17, 37, 52–6
   Flowtron machine 129
   frequency of treatment 53
   hydrotherapy 62–3
   importance of persevering
      56
   and occupational therapy
      141
   over-eagerness to exercise
      54–5
   therapist's role and training
      52, 53–4
platelets 7, 163, 166, 227*g*, 231*g*
Plavix (clopidogrel) 34, 168,
   169
polypill 171
positron emission tomography
   (PET) 224, 231*g*
power of attorney 220
pravastatin 77
pregnancy 163, 201–2
pressure sores 31, 38, 65,
   105–7
prochlorperazine (Stemetil)
   137
progesterone 160

prognosis 11, 15, 231*g*
pronunciation *see* dyspraxia
propranolol 165
prostaglandin 198
Prozac (fluoxetine) 114, 116
psychological problems *19*,
   109–10
pulmonary embolism 231*g*
pulse 159

quinine 128

race factor and risk 157, 165,
   224
ramipril 164
ranitidine 34
REACT computer program 95
reading difficulties 134, 227*g*
recombinant tissue
   plasminogen activator
   (rtPA) 29–30
recovery after stroke 13–15,
   17, 19–20
rectum 104
Red Cross equipment 65, 143
reflex sympathetic dystrophy
   129
rehabilitation issues 38–50,
   231*g*
   at home 40, 178, 181–2
   being overweight 84
   degree of intensity 48
   in hospital 40–8
   psychological problems
      109–10
   when to start 38–9, 63
   *see also individual
      treatments*

relationships 156, 195–6
  sexual matters 114, 196–201
    erection problems 197–8
    female orgasm 200–1
    positioning 199
  vaginal dryness 201
relaxation techniques 124
repetition of words 90–1
research 1
  carotid endarterectomy 172
  future developments 221–5
  genetic factors 157
  growth hormone 61
  taking part in studies 222
  value of stroke units 40–1
  see also clinical trials
residential home see care
    home
respite care 204–7
  see also care home; carers
retina of eye 133
rheumatoid arthritis 162
risk factors 147, 231g
  Afro-Caribbean people 157,
    165, 224
  anger 156
  contraceptive pill 160–1
  diabetes 160
  from surgery 173
  heart disease 157–8
  heart murmurs 156–7
  heredity 147–8
  high blood pressure 148–50
  HRT 161
  irregular heart rhythm 158–9
  smoking 150–3
  snoring 159–60
  stress 153–5

TIAs 155–6
  in young people 161–2
rtPA (recombinant tissue
    plasminogen activator)
    29–30

safety problems 45–6, 141–2
saliva 123, 176
salt 79–80, 150
scapula 55, 125
scooters, electric 66
seizure see epilepsy
selective serotonin re-uptake
    inhibitors (SSRIs) 114
senna 103
sensation 122, 129–31, 200
  see also hemi-neglect
senses 132
Serc (betahistine) 137
sertraline 114
sexual matters see
    relationships, sexual
    matters
shellfish 77
sheltered housing 186–7
shock 153
shoulder problems 55, 125
shunt (surgical) 35
sickle cell disease 163
sight see vision
simvastatin 77, 171
singing 90
sinus problems 126
skills see activities of daily
    living
skin care 104–7
skin problems 98
  see also sensation

sleep problems 18, 118–21, 159
smell and taste 136
smoking 151–3
snoring 159–60
social services 178–80, 182,
    184, 186
  care homes 182, 184, 187–9
  respite care 205–6
sodium in urine 164
sodium valproate (Epilim) 176
sotalol 165
spasticity 57, 128, 231*g*
specialists (medical) 37–8, 156
speech problems 10, 36, 86–92
  aphasia 115, 228*g*
  bilingual 88–9
  communication aids 94–5
  dysarthria 89, 94, 229*g*
  dysphasia 86–8, 92–3, 94,
    229*g*
  dyspraxia 89, 94, 229*g*
  and music 90
  perseveration 90–1
  questioning 94
  therapy 29, 37, 88–9, 92–5
    how much/how long
      needed 92–3
  voice changes 91, 113
splinting of limbs 59
sports 127, 154, 212–14
SSRIs (selective serotonin
    re-uptake inhibitors) 114
statistics
  age and incidence 43–4
  aneurysm repair 174
  aspirin vs warfarin 169
  causes of strokes 7, 8
  death rates 30

epilepsy and stroke 175, 176
incidence 1
incontinence in women 99
recovery of normal vision
    133
return to normality 14
risk with thrombolysis 30
stroke management 42
stroke resulting from
    surgery 173
treatment of central post-
    stroke pain 123
Stemetil (prochlorperazine)
    137
stenosis 157, 231*g*
steroids 60–1, 125
stockings, anti-thrombosis 32
stomach ulcers 34, 170
streptokinase 29
stress 153–5
stroke
  causes 11, 161–2
  haemorrhagic 8, 9–10, 214
  ischaemic 33
  mini-stroke (lacunar) 9,
    230*g*
  more than one 15–16, 18
  prevention 84–5
  recovery process 13–15, 17,
    18, 56, 181–2, 224
  silent 11
  similar symptoms *19*
  symptoms and early care 30
  warning signs 174–5
  what it is 6–8, *7*
  see also drugs; home care;
    hospital care;
    occupational therapy;

stroke: *see also (continued)*
   personal care; physio-
     therapy; rehabilitation
     issues; risk factors;
     surgery; swallowing;
     treatment
Stroke Association 216, 225
subdural haematoma 18, *19*
subluxation 55
support groups 191
suppositories 104
surgery
   for brain swelling 34, 35
   carotid angioplasty 173–4
   carotid endarterectomy 26,
     172–3
   cutting tendons 59
   hip/knee replacement 127–8
   resulting in stroke 173
   to prevent stroke 172–4
swallowing
   and nutrition 68–9
   problems 28–9, 36, 39,
     69–75
   recovery rate 73
swelling
   ankle 165
   brain 17, 34, 118–19
   face and throat 167
   hand 128–9
swimming 81–2, 213
systemic lupus erythematosus
   (SLE) 162

taste and smell 136
teeth care 69
Tegretol (carbamazepine) 123,
   176

telephone use 180
temperature of body 35
TENS *see* transcutaneous
   electrical nerve
   stimulation
tests 23–9
   see also individual tests:
     e.g. carotid doppler
thalamus 123, 231*g*
throat investigation 27–8
thrombolysis 29–30, 232*g*
thrombosis 32, 232*g*
thrush 104–5
TIA *see* transient ischaemic
   attack
tingling sensation 129
tiredness *see* fatigue
tissue plasminogen activator
   (tPA) 29, 223, 232*g*
tizanidine 58, 128
tolterodine 101
tPA *see* tissue plasminogen
   activator
trachea 69
transcutaneous electrical
   nerve stimulation (TENS)
   124, 129
transient ischaemic attack
   (TIA) 8–9, 230*g*, 232*g*
   tests required 155–6
travel 213, 214–15
treatment
   brain swelling 34
   central post-stroke pain
     123–4
   getting moving 51
   private 36–7, 48–9
   prolonging life 21–2

subarachnoid haemorrhage
36
see also complementary
therapies; drugs; home
care; hospital care;
physiotherapy; surgery
tumour of brain 18, *19*, 126

ultrasound examination 26, 71,
155, 172
understanding, problems in
87–8
urethra 198
urinary problems 97–103
catheter 98–9, 196–7, 228*g*
infection 100, 101–2
retention of urine 98–9, 114
sodium in urine 164

vagina 201
Valium (diazepam) 128
valsartan 164
vasculitis 162
ventricular septal defect 157,
232*g*
vertigo 137, 232*g*
Viagra 198–9
video-fluoroscopy 29
vision 66, 133–6, 229*g*
double 135–6, 216
hemianopia 133, 135, 230*g*
loss as warning sign 175
reading difficulties 134
visual neglect 135
vitamins 74, 85
voice *see* speech problems
Voltarol (diclofenac) 125

walking 7, 51, 54, 58
after hospital discharge
181–2
for pleasure 212
unsteadiness as warning
sign 175
walking frame vs stick 61–2,
127
warfarin 158, 169–70, 232*g*
not to be combined with
aspirin 170
see also aspirin
warning signs of stroke
174–5
water tablets *see* diuretics
weakness in limbs 175
weeping 116
weight
body mass index 82–3, *83*
loss after stroke 73–4
overweight (obesity) 75–6,
80–3, 84, 150, 231*g*
wheelchairs 64–6, 142, 143–4
windpipe (oesophagus) 27–8,
69
work 153–5, 215–17
writing difficulties 93–4

X-ray *see* arteriogram;
computed tomography
(CT) scan; magnetic
resonance imaging (MRI);
ultrasound examination;
video-fluoroscopy

yoga 124, 154

zinc deficiency 136

The *'At Your Fingertips'* guide Feedback Form

We hope that you found this *'at your fingertips'* guide helpful. We always appreciate readers' opinions and would be grateful if you could take a few minutes to complete this form for us.

1 **How did you acquire your copy of this book?**

From my local library ☐

Read an article in a newspaper/magazine ☐

Found it by chance ☐

Recommended by a friend ☐

Recommended by a patient organisation/charity ☐

Recommended by a doctor/nurse/advisor ☐

Saw an advertisement ☐

2 **How much of the book have you read?**

All of it ☐

More than half of it ☐

Less than half of it ☐

3 **Which copies/chapters have been most helpful?**

....

....

4 **Overall, how useful to you was this *'at your fingertips'* guide?**

Extremely useful ☐

Very useful ☐

Useful ☐

5 **What did you find most helpful?**

....

....

❻ What did you find least helpful?

....

....

❼ Have you read any other health books?

Yes ☐   No ☐

If yes, which subjects did they cover?

....

....

How did this 'at your fingertips' guide compare?

Much better   ☐

Better   ☐

About the same   ☐

Not as good   ☐

❽ Would you recommend this book to a friend?

Yes ☐   No ☐

Thank you for your help. Please send your completed form to:

Class Publishing, FREEPOST, London W6 7BR

Surname   First name

Title Prof/Dr/Mr/Mrs/Ms

Address

Town   Postcode   Country

☐ Please add my name and address to receive details of related books
[*Please note, we will not pass on your details to any other company*]

Have you found **Stroke – the 'at your fingertips' guide** useful and practical? If so, you may be interested in other books from Class Publishing.

Stop that heart attack!   £14.99
Dr Derrick Cutting

The easy, drug-free and medically accurate way to cut dramatically your risk of having a heart attack. Even if you already have heart disease, you can halt and even reverse its progress by following Dr Cutting's simple steps. Don't be a victim – take action NOW!

'This is an exceptional book.' – *Cardiology News*

Heart Health – the 'at your fingertips' guide   £17.99
NEW FOURTH EDITION
Dr Graham Jackson

This practical handbook, written by a leading cardiologist, answers all your questions about heart conditions. It tells you all about you and your heart; how to keep your heart healthy – or, if it has been affected by heart disease, how to make it as strong as possible.

'Those readers who want to know more about the various treatments for heart disease will be much enlightened.'
– Dr James Le Fanu, *The Daily Telegraph*

Diabetes – the 'at your fingertips' guide   £14.99
Professor Peter Sönksen, Dr Charles Fox and Sue Judd

This is an invaluable reference guide for people with diabetes, which offers practical advice on every aspect of living with the condition, giving you the knowledge and reassurance you need to deal confidently with your diabetes.

'I have no hesitation in commending this book.'
– Sir Steve Redgrave CBE, Vice President, Diabetes UK

High Blood Pressure – the 'at your fingertips' guide £14.99
Professor Tom Fahey, Professor Deirdre Murphy
with Dr Julian Tudor Hart

The authors use all their years of experience as blood pressure experts to answer your questions on high blood pressure, in order to give you the information you need to bring your blood pressure down – and keep it down.

'Readable and comprehensive information'
– Dr Sylvia McLaughlan, Director General,
The Stroke Association

**Dementia: Alzheimer's and other dementias – the
'at your fingertips' guide** £14.99
Harry Cayton, Dr Nori Graham and Dr James Warner

This fully revised and updated book outlines the different care options that are available and suggests a variety of strategies for coping with dementia. It tells people where to go for help and guidance on legal, financial and other matters and gives advice on how to prepare for the future and make difficult decisions.

'This book cannot be recommended too highly.'
– Claire Rayner, *Mail on Sunday*

Beating Depression £17.99
Dr Stefan Cembrowicz and Dr Dorcas Kingham

Depression is one of most common illnesses in the world – affecting up to one in four people at some time in their lives. *Beating Depression* shows sufferers and their families that they are not alone, and offers tried and tested techniques for overcoming depression.

PRIORITY ORDER FORM

Cut out or photocopy this form and send it (post free in the UK) to:

Class Publishing Priority Service
FREEPOST
London W6 7BR

Please send me urgently   Post included
(tick boxes below)   price per copy *(UK only)*

☐ **Stroke – the 'at your fingertips' guide** (ISBN 1 85959 113 2)   £20.99

☐ **Stop that heart attack!** (ISBN 1 85959 096 9)   £17.99

☐ **Heart Health – the 'at your fingertips' guide** (ISBN 1 85959 157 4)   £20.99

☐ **Diabetes – the 'at your fingertips' guide** (ISBN 1 85959 087 X)   £17.99

☐ **High Blood Pressure – the 'at your fingertips' guide**   £17.99
(ISBN 1 85959 090 X)

☐ **Dementia: Alzheimer's and other dementias**
– the 'at your fingertips' guide (ISBN 1 85959 075 6)   £17.99

☐ **Beating Depression** (ISBN 1 85959 150 7)   £20.99

TOTAL _____

EASY WAYS TO PAY

Cheque: I enclose a cheque payable to Class Publishing for £ _____

Credit card: Please debit my   ☐ Mastercard   ☐ Visa   ☐ Amex

Number _____   Expiry date ___ / ___

Name _____

My address for delivery is _____

_____

Town _____ County _____ Postcode _____

Telephone number *(in case of query)* _____

Credit card billing address *(if different from above)* _____

_____

Town _____ County _____ Postcode _____

Class Publishing's guarantee: remember that if, for any reason, you are not satisfied with these books, we will refund all your money, without any questions asked. Prices and VAT rates may be altered for reasons beyond our control.